This work: "X-Ray Contrast Media: Overview, Use and Pharmaceutical Aspects",
was originally published by Springer Nature and is being sold pursuant to a
Creative Commons license permitting commercial use. All rights not granted by
the work's license are retained by the author or authors.

*Cover Image Credit/Copyright Attribution: IIIerlok_Xolms/Shutterstock*

Ulrich Speck

# X-Ray Contrast Media

## Overview, Use and Pharmaceutical Aspects

5. Auflage

Ulrich Speck
InnoRa GmbH
Berlin, Germany

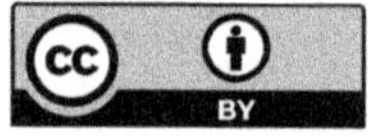

https://doi.org/10.1007/978-3-662-56465-3



This Open Access is sponsored by Bayer AG, Berlin

# CONTENT

# INTRODUCTION

## Historical Aspects

The field of radiography including the development of contrast media for this diagnostic tool is based on the discovery of X-rays by the physicist Wilhelm Conrad Röntgen. Later on, the rays he discovered came to be called "Roentgen rays" in his honor.

Experimenting with electrons Röntgen observed effects he attributed to so-called cathode rays, hitherto unknown rays, which he called "X-rays". To prove his ideas and the penetration of different kinds of matter by this new type of radiation, Röntgen used a fluoroscope and a photographic plate. On December 22, 1895, he succeeded in taking a picture of the bones of his wife's hand using X-rays.

Röntgen assumed his newly discovered rays to be electromagnetic radiation like visible light. In April 1912, this assumption was confirmed by the physicist Max von Laue and his coworkers. The wave-like behavior of X-rays was proven by the detection of diffraction and interference patterns produced by X-rays transmitted through crystals.

Physicians all over the world soon recognized the diagnostic potential of Röntgen's discovery. The new rays gave physicians the ability to see inside the body and obtain pictures not only of bones and soft tissues but also of hollow organs by using radiopaque substances. In 1896, barium sulfate (BaSO4) was used for the first time to examine intestinal peristalsis, a procedure which was soon to fall into oblivion again. Only ten years later, the so-called Rieder meal (barium mixed with gruel) was introduced for X-ray examinations of the gastrointestinal tract.

© The Author(s) 2018

U. Speck, *X-Ray Contrast Media*, https://doi.org/10.1007/978-3-662-56465-3_1

While the ability of iodine to absorb X-rays was discovered as early as 1896, it took almost another thirty years to develop the first X-ray contrast medium (XCM) for clinical use. The oily iodine compound Lipiodol was introduced as the first reliable X-ray contrast agent for myelography. In 1924, the first oral biliary XCM, Iodtetragnost (iodophthalein) for visualization of the gallbladder was put on the market. This was followed by the introduction of less toxic cholecystographic XCM like Biliselectan (iodoalphionic acid) in 1940 and later on the more tolerable Biloptin (sodium iopodate). In 1953, Biligrafin (adipiodone) was established as the first i.v. XCM for visualizing the gallbladder and biliary tract in the routine diagnostic setting. Further development led to another two well-tolerable XCM – Endomirabil (iodoxamic acid) and Biliscopin (iotroxic acid) – agents that are mostly used in cholecystocholoangiography.

Uroselectan was the first reliable urographic contrast agent. It is a water-soluble organic iodine compound that is excreted via the kidneys and entered the market in 1929. Concomitantly, the long line of soluble XCM with iodinated pyridine rings and later on with benzene rings began.

In the early 1950s, there was a rapid switch from diiodinated pyridine derivates to benzene derivates with three iodine atoms, the tri-ioidinated benzoic acid.

Hydrophilic side groups as well as methylglucamine, which is used for salt formation, significantly improved the tolerance of ionic XCM.

In the late 1960s, the significance of hyperosmolality but also that of electric charge as causes of specific adverse effects of ionic XCM became clear. Almen's suggestion to replace the ionic carboxyl group in tri-iodinated benzoic acid derivates with a non dissociated group, i.e. a carbohydrate, and to ensure the necessary water solubility by utilizing particularly hydrophilic hydroxyl groups marks the beginning of nonionic XCM. The latest advancement of X-ray contrast agents led to the hexa-iodinated, nonionic dimers Iotrolan and Iodixanol, which have the same osmolality as blood and cerebrospinal fluid at all concentrations.

The initial expectation that iso-osmolality would further improve the side effect profile has not been confirmed in clinical studies. Therefore, the tri-iodinated monomeric nonionic contrast media remain the workhorse in contrast-enhanced X-ray examinations.

Nonionic monomeric or dimeric X-ray contrast media are applied in all areas of diagnostic radiology.

In addition to the positive XCM mentioned so far, negative XCM such as air, oxygen and carbon dioxide, which absorb X-rays less well than biological tissues, are applied for visualizing hollow organs. The use of negative XCM has become rare with the advent of sophisticated imaging modalities such as CT and MRI.

## Contrast media in X-ray imaging

The significance of contrast media was recognized almost simultaneously with the discovery of X-rays. Too many structures in the body remain invisible when X-rays alone are used and can only be made visible after administration of a contrast medium.

As a result, much effort has been spent to better adapt contrast agents and the techniques of their administration to diagnostic requirements and to improve their tolerability.

At the same time, imaging technologies have continued to develop, and computed tomography and subtraction techniques improve the contrast resolution of X-ray images. However, contrast media still have their uses with new imaging modalities as well.

**Visualization of functions**
- elimination (kidney, liver)
- transport processes (bloodstream, cerebrospinal fluid, intestinal contents, imaging of the liver)
- perfusion (all organs)
- permeability and barriers (blood-brain barrier, cysts)

**Morphology**
- Creating and increasing contrasts, for example, through
    - varying contrast media concentrations in individual tissues
    - temporal changes of radiation absorption or signal intensities

On the whole, all imaging techniques and all products referred to as contrast media have one thing in common – they all assist in providing visual representations of information from within the body.

This information may represent anatomical structures, functions, or physical-chemical conditions.

# GENERAL PRINCIPLES OF X-RAY CONTRAST MEDIA

Contrast in an X-ray image is brought about by differences in absorption of X-rays by the tissues being irradiated. Absorption is dependent on the atomic number of the atoms present in the molecules, the concentration of these molecules and the thickness of the irradiated slice. When a chest radiograph is obtained , the bones, the aeriferous lungs, the heart and other tissues provide adequate natural contrast. In other body regions such as the abdomen, however, the composition of the organs is so similar that the differences in absorption are too small and other measures are required to enhance the differences in absorption and make the organs visible;  (fig. 1). The introduction of substances of very low density (gases) into organs or surrounding structures reduces absorption, and such substances are called negative contrast media (CM). Substances with a high X-ray density contain atoms of higher atomic numbers (barium or iodine). Such preparations increase the absorption of X-rays in the body and are, therefore, known as positive CM (table 1)

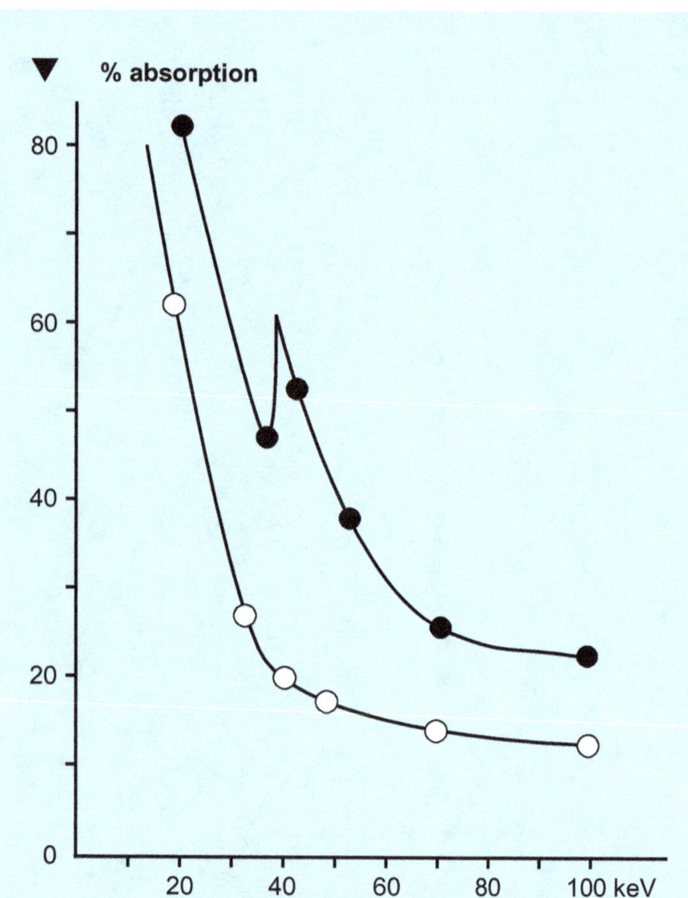


**Fig. 1.** Absorption of X-rays in % by water (~ soft tissue, ◯–◯) and an aqueous CM solution with 20 mg iodine/ml (●–●) with slice thickness of 1 cm in relation to the energy of the X-rays (50 keV are achieved at about 100 kV tube voltage)



U. Speck, *X-Ray Contrast Media*, https://doi.org/10.1007/978-3-662-56465-3_2

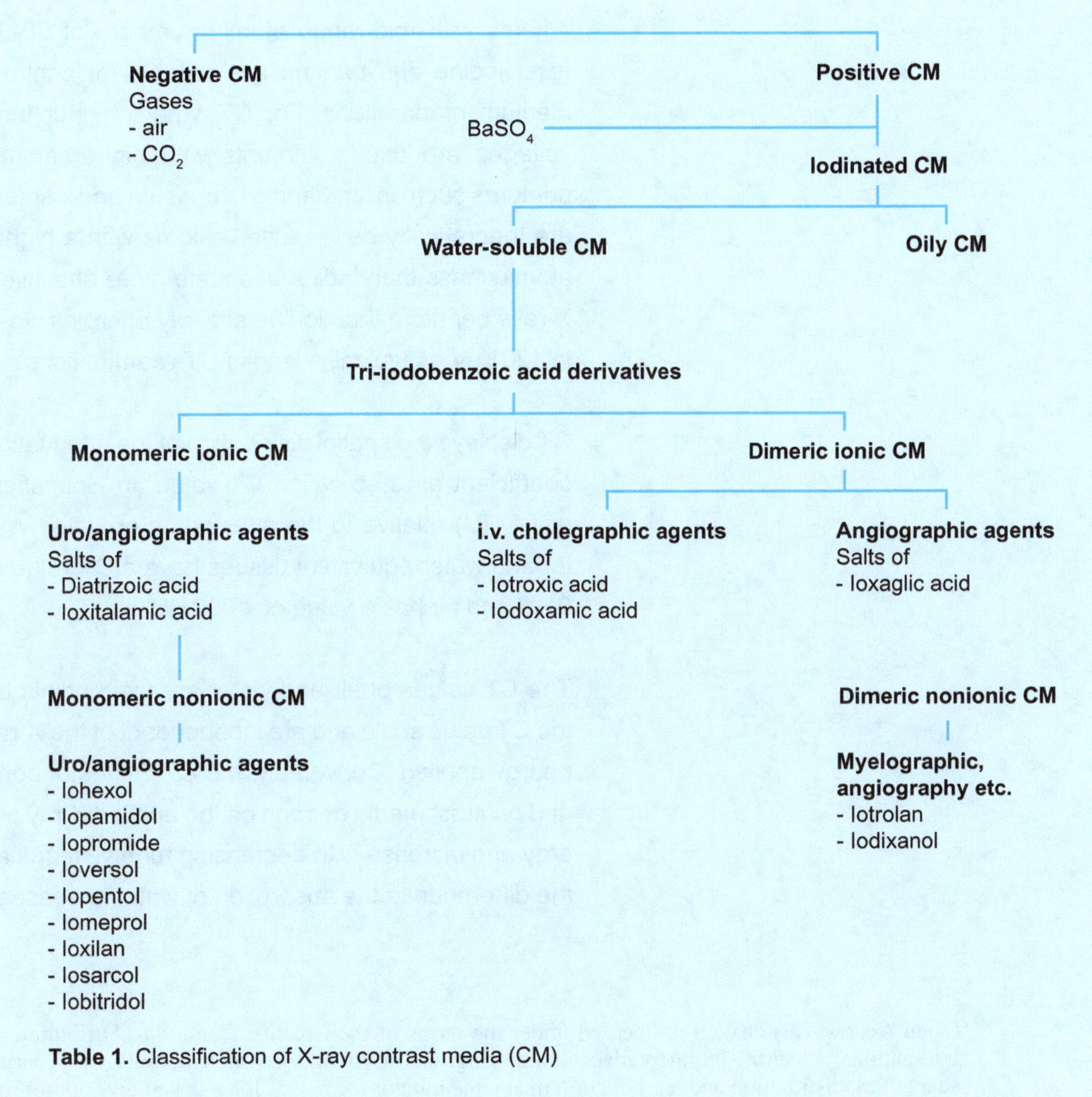


**Table 1.** Classification of X-ray contrast media (CM)

## Physical Principles

Contrast medium absorption primarily depends on the mass absorption coefficient of the elements present in the molecules and applied the X-ray energy spectrum. Secondarily, it also depends on the concentration of these molecules in the tissues. Elements with mid-range atomic numbers of 50-60 (e.g., iodine and barium) are suitable for contrast medium preparations. For CT, where higher tube voltages are used, elements with higher atomic numbers such as lanthanoids, tungsten and bismuth are theoretically better suited. Atoms with a higher atomic mass than iodine attenuate more effectively X-rays per atom than iodine at X-ray energies close to 120 KeV as typically used in CT examinations.

CT displays the spatial distribution of the attenuation coefficient as a so-called CT value (in Hounsfield units, HU) relative to the attenuation of water. Water and water-equivalent tissues have a CT value of 0 HU and air has a value of -1000 HU.

The CT values of air and water are fixed points on the CT value scale and are independent of the X-ray energy applied. Conversely, the CT values of bone and contrast media depend on the applied X-ray energy and increase with decreasing tube voltages as the difference to the absorption of water increases.



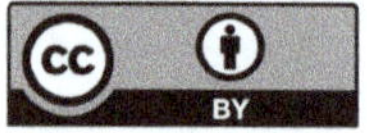

# STRUCTURE AND PROPERTIES OF X-RAY CONTRAST MEDIA

Optimal use of CM in radiology requires a knowledge of the nature and relevant properties of the available substances. This chapter describes the properties of currently used and newly developed contrast-giving agents that influence their behavior in the human body, their side effects, and their practical utility.

The main X-ray contrast agents in use today are insoluble barium sulfate for the diagnostic evaluation of the GI tract and water-soluble CM for the radiological assessment of the different vascular systems, body cavities and organs. In addition, a water-soluble CM based on tri-iodobenzene is the alternative agent of choice for oral use when barium sulfate is contraindicated.

## Barium Sulfate

Barium is used in the form of the insoluble sulfate for radiography of the GI tract. If perforation is suspected, however, only water-soluble, iodinated agents (Gastrografin, Ultravist-370) can be used since the body is virtually incapable of eliminating barium sulfate once it has entered the peritoneum. Barium sulfate is available either as a powder to be prepared directly before use or as a ready-to-use suspension. For double-contrast examinations (filling of the lumen with gas, coating of the wall with barium sulfate), barium sulfate is either mixed with a carbon dioxide additive, or a gas-forming agent is taken in addition.


U. Speck, *X-Ray Contrast Media*, https://doi.org/10.1007/978-3-662-56465-3_3

Common to all barium preparations is concentration of barium sulfate which may diluted according to the needs of the examination. The amount of suspension needed depends on the type of examination and the target organ to be examined [1].

## Lipiodol

Lipiodol and other iodinated herbal oils have been in use for a wide range of different purposes, including myelography, ventriculography, hysterosalpingography and lymphography, since the beginning of radiology, mainly due to their low acute local toxicity. Lipiodol used to be the most popular compound made of poppyseed oil, whose unsaturated fatty acids were substituted with iodine.

The iodinated oils that are in use today are mono-, di- and tri-iodinated ethyl esters of a mixture of various saturated and unsatured fatty acids in poppyseed oil as carrier (Lipiodol UF, Ethiodol). Those highly fluid and better-tolerated substances are or were used for visualization of fine structures in direct lymphography, for hysterosalpingography and mixed with cyanoacrylate for embolization of endoleaks.

In addition, Lipiodol mixed with cytostatic agents (e.g., doxorubicin) can be used for the treatment of hepatocellular carcinoma (HCC), because iodine-lipids embolize the vasculature and to some extent accumulate in cancer cells.

Liver lesions as small as 2 mm can be made visible in a CT scan. In a study of 47 patients examined by CT after intra-arterial Lipiodol, 5-10 ml of Lipiodol mixed with chemotherapeutic agents and a water-soluble CM was infused via a catheter whose tip was advanced into a hepatic artery, either into the common hepatic artery or selectively into the right or left hepatic artery. Lipiodol-CT was statistically superior to sonography, CT and angiography in detecting small hepatocellular carcinomas [2]. The exact mechanism of this accumulation remains unclear. The selective intra-arterial injection of Lipiodol combined with a cytostatic agent (e.g., doxorubicin) into hepatic artery branches that supply a hepatic tumor is known as transarterial chemoembolization (TACE) and is used to induce tumor necrosis by slowly releasing the trapped cytostatic agent from Lipiodol-embolized tissue.

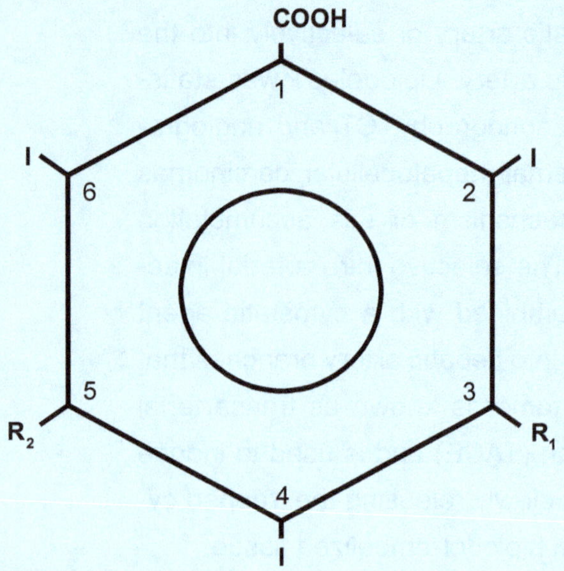

**Fig. 2.** Structure of tri-iodinated CM
Aromate = Parent substance
-COOH = Salt or amide binding, water solubility
-I = Contrast-giving component
-R₁ R₂ = Reduction of toxity and lipophilia
-R₂ = Elimination pathway

## Water-soluble contrast media

The first CM on the basis of ionic tri-iodobenzene were introduced around 1950 (fig. 2) and had virtually taken over the field by the second half of the fifties. In the 1980s, the ionic forms were largely replaced by CM on the basis of non-ionic tri-iodobenzene. The reasons why such a homogeneous substance class still dominates intravascular contrast medium applications in X-ray-based radiological examinations without any recognizable competition are as follows:

- Iodine is the only chemical element which combines three properties essential for the production of a successful CM: high contrast density, chemical behavior which allows firm binding to the highly variable benzene molecule, and low toxicity.
- The iodine is optimally bound in the symmetrically substituted tri-iodobenzene; at 84 %, the iodine content of the basic molecule is extremely high.
- Positions 1, 3 and 5 in the molecule are available to the chemist for the most diverse modifications of the physicochemical and biological properties by the introduction of side chains.

**Chemical structure, biological behavior and use**
The substance classes shown in figure 3 were produced by varying the basic molecule of tri-iodobenzene. Thanks to the large variety of substances that were synthesized, the relationship between the chemical structure of the molecules and their principal biological behavior is well documented.

## High-osmolar, ionic contrast media

Diatrizoic acid, which was introduced in 1953, is contained in numerous products and was the most widely used CM in the world for urography, angiography and CT for three decades. Because its COOH group is connected directly to the tri-iodobenzene ring, diatrizoic acid (Urografin, Angiografin, Urovist, Urovison) is a strong acid, forming salts which are readily soluble in water. The two side chains ($-NHCOCH_3$) further improve the solubility, reduce protein binding (thereby increasing its ability to be filtered in the glomerulus) and improve above all the tolerance. The substance is eliminated almost exclusively via the kidneys. There is a series of related compounds which are derived from diatrizoic acid; meanwhile, however, these are less important. Nowadays, the use of high-osmolar ionic contrast media decreases due to better tolerance and same efficacy of low-osmolar nonionic CM. However, ionic CM still matters as an oral CM and in radiological examinations of body cavities.

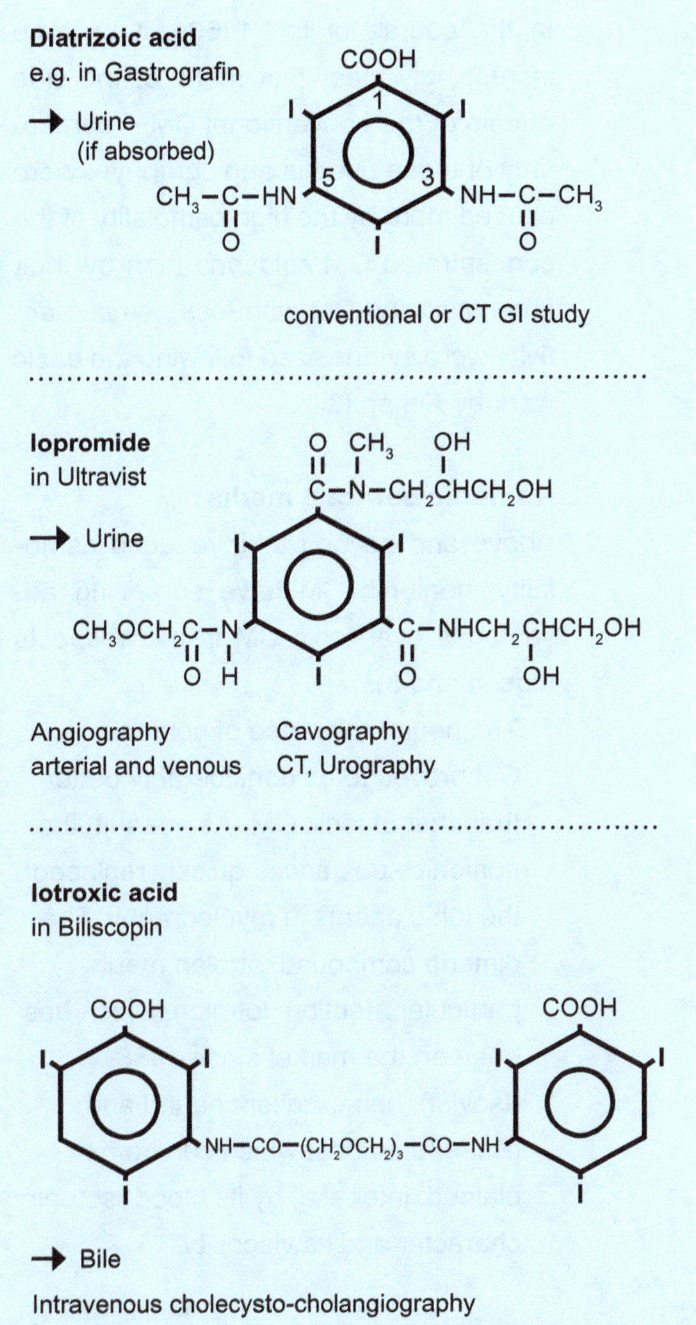


Fig. 3: Basic chemical structures of water-soluble CM, main elimination pathway, fields of use as exemplified by a representative of each substance class

**Low-osmolar substances**

In the course of the 1960s, it became increasingly clear that many of the side effects of the conventional CM – particularly of those used in angiography – were caused more by the high osmolality of the concentrated CM solutions than by their chemotoxicity. CM with less osmotic activity were synthesized following the basic work by Almén [3].

**Nonionic contrast media**

Above and beyond their reduced osmolality, nonionic CM have surprising advantages over ionic CM in two respects (figs. 4 and 5):

1. The neural tolerance of nonionic CM proved to be considerably better than that of ionic CM. As a result, the nonionic substances quickly replaced the ionic agents in myelography. The dimeric compound iotrolan merits particular mention. Iotrolan, which has been on the market since 1988 (Isovist), has excellent neural and tissue tolerance, which can be explained, inter alia, by its blood-isotonic character and its viscosity.

2. The incidence of both general reactions, such as nausea and vomiting, and of the sometimes life-threatening, acute allergy-like or idiosyncratic reactions, is apparently far lower when nonionic CM are given [4, 5, 6, 7, 8, 9].

As a result more than 90 % of ionic CM in angiography, urography and CT have been replaced by nonionic products today. However, the incidence of fatal reactions is too rare to allow statistical comparison. The good general tolerance of nonionic CM compared to that of ionic CM and the low-osmolar compound ioxaglate can be explained by the following main properties:

Nonionic contrast media
- contain no electrical charges,
- contain no cations, such as sodium or meglumine, and
- are considerably better shielded by hydrophilic side chains.

This results in minimal protein binding and enzyme inhibition and in reduced impairment of the function of biological membranes.

For the patient, this means substantially better general tolerance. Nausea and vomiting, urticaria, mucosal swelling, increased respiratory resistance and effects on the cardiovascular system are less frequently observed with nonionic CM.

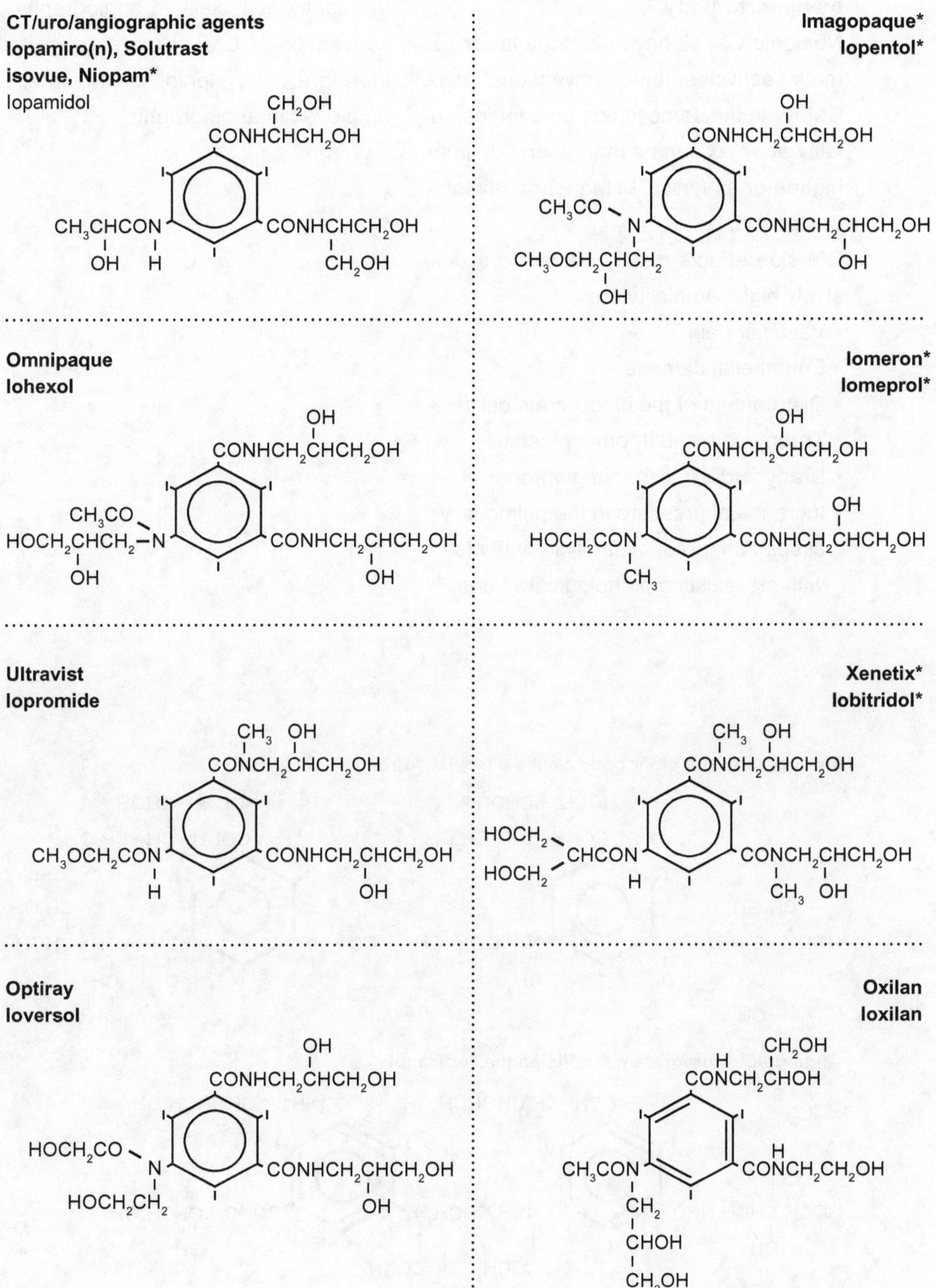

**Fig. 4.** Chemical structures of nonionic CM for angiography, urography and CT

**Osmolality and side effects caused by hypertonicity**

Nonionic CM all have distinctly lower osmotic activities than conventional ionic CM. With the same iodine content, osmolality at 37° C can be more than 2.5 times higher for an ionic CM than for a nonionic compound.

CM side effects mainly related to excessively high osmolality are:

• Vascular pain
• Endothelial damage
• Disturbance of the blood-brain barrier
• Thrombosis and thrombophlebitis
• Bradycardia in cardioangiography
• Increase of pressure in the pulmonary circulation, predominantly in patients with pre-existing pathological values.

Some of these side effects occur very frequently especially in angiography with conventional CM. Wherever possible, therefore, only nonionic CM should be employed in angiography.

**Myelography and other body cavities: Isovist, Iotrolan**

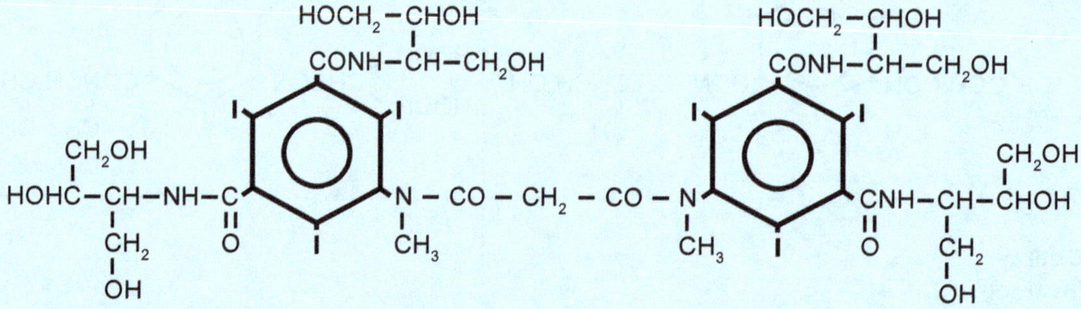

**Angiography, urography, CT: Visipaque, Iodixanol**

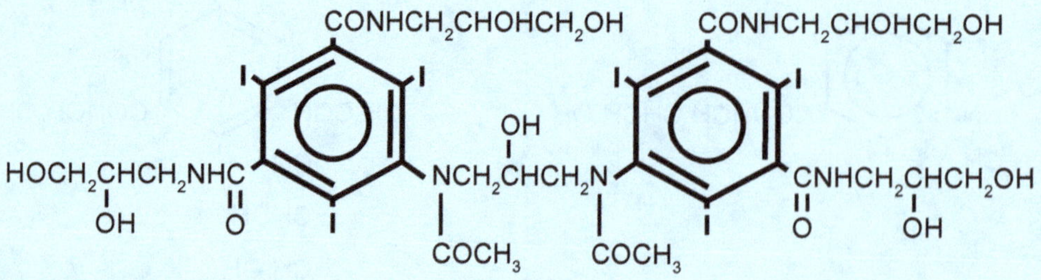

**Fig. 5.** Chemical structures of nonionic dimeric X-ray CM

| | Osmolality 300 mg l/ml, 37°C mosm/kg $H_2O$ mean and 95% confidence interval | Viscosity, 37°C | | Protein binding in % at 1.2 mg l/ml plasma |
| --- | --- | --- | --- | --- |
| | | 300 mg l/ml m Pa · s | 370 mg l/ml m Pa · s | |
| Iopromide | 586 ± 5 | 4.6 | 9.5 | 0.9 ± 0.2 |
| Iopamidol | 653 ± 7 | 4.5 | 9.5 | 2.9 ± 0.2 |
| Iohexol | 667 ± 8 | 5.7 | 10.5* | 1.5 ± 0.3 |
| Ioversol | 661 ± 3 | 5.5 | 9.0* | 1.6 ± 0.9** |
| Iopentol | 683 ± 4 | 6.5 | 12.0* | 1.9 ± 0.6*** |
| Iomeprol | 538 | 4.3 | 7.0* | 1.7 ± 0.4 |
| Iobitridol | 695 | 6.0 | 10.0* | - |

* 350 mg Iod/ml       ** more than Iopromide       *** less than Iohexol

**Table 2.** Nonionic CM for intravascular administration

At high dosage and irrespective of the mode of administration, high-osmolality CM cause general vasodilatation and a drop in blood pressure, hypervolemia and diuresis. When nonionic CM are used, these effects are less severe or only occur at an even higher dosage.

How do nonionic CM differ from each other?

Nonionic CM differ (because of their chemical structure) in terms of their osmolality, their viscosity, and their substance-specific properties. Comparative measurements were performed. The results are presented in tables 2 and 3 [10]. When an individual nonionic CM for a given purpose is chosen taking into account its specific properties, radiodiagnosis can be optimized and the risk for the patient reduced.

| | Osmolality mosm/kg $H_2O$ | Viscosity m Pa · s, 37°C |
| --- | --- | --- |
| Iotrolan | | |
| Isovist-240 | 270 | 3.9 |
| Isovist-300 | 291 | 8.1 |
| Iopamidol-200 | 413 | 2.0 |
| Iopamidol-250 | 580 | 3.0 |
| Iohexol-180 | 390 | 2.0 |
| Iohexol-240 | 520 | 3.3 |

**Table 3.** Nonionic CM for myelography and other body cavities (Isovist)

### Ionic contrast media

It is also possible to produce low-osmolar ionic CM. The only one of these CM to have achieved any importance in angiography is meglumine sodium ioxaglate (Hexabrix [11]). Its use is confined to angiography because it has neither the neural nor the general tolerance of nonionic CM [12, 13].

Ioxaglate (Hexabrix, only one acid function) consists of two tri-iodobenzene rings (dimers) which are connected via a chain (fig. 6).

The resulting doubling of the molecular weight has no influence on the basic properties of the molecules: Good solubility, renal elimination and a lack of enteral absorption suggest the same uses as for diatrizoate. The distinctly lower osmotic pressure of sodium meglumine ioxaglate solutions is why patients experience virtually no pain after administration for peripheral angiography. High viscosity and a higher rate of general reactions are disadvantages of ioxaglate.

**Ioxaglate**

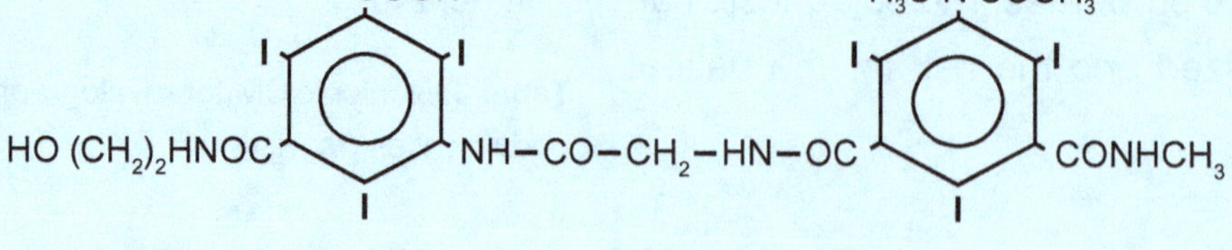

**Fig. 6.** Monocarbonic acid dimer

**Contrast media for intravenous cholegraphy**

As for urography, CM with very similar chemical properties are available for i.v. cholegraphy. Unlike the urographic agents, however, not every i.v. cholegraphic agent has its specific advantages and disadvantages, since it was possible to improve the first i.v. cholegraphic agent, iodipamide, in terms of both opacification and tolerance.

Iodipamide (Biligrafin) is the prototypical i.v. biliary CM. It is a dimeric diacid which contains no further side chains. It is eliminated for the greater part with the bile without the molecules undergoing any chemical changes (metabolism).

The modern i.v. biliary CM Biliscopin is bound somewhat less firmly to albumin. The rate of elimination and the contrast density are increased; tolerance is very much improved, especially when the CM is administered by infusion. Since a constant infusion rate is decisive for tolerance the use of an automatic infusion pump is recommended.

**Cations**

The ionic CM for angiography, urography, CT, i.v. cholegraphy and oral cholegraphy are sufficiently soluble in water only as salts. While, for most oral biliary CM, the formation of salt is left to the organism, a few oral cholegraphic agents and all the other compounds mentioned are offered as finished salts. Iodine-free bases (usually sodium or meglumine) are used to dissolve the iodinated CM acid.

At present, diatrizoate is also available as a lysine salt only in Germany and ioxithalamate as an ethanolamine (mixed) salt only in France. Numerous other cations can be used as counterions for CM acids but, so far, no cations have been found which are better suited than or even as well as meglumine or sodium.

The cations introduced into the body with the CM are freely mobile independently of the CM acids and are eliminated independently of the acids.

As far as is known at present, the pharmacokinetics of the acids are not affected by the cations [14, 15]. Similar to the CM anion, the meglumine cation diffuses into the extracellular space with only little uptake into cells and is eliminated almost exclusively via the kidneys. Sodium behaves the same as endogenous sodium. Meglumine, which was originally introduced because of the solubility of its salts, has, in general, proved to be a well tolerated cation.

Disadvantages of meglumine are the higher viscosity and the somewhat stronger diuretic effect. A certain proportion of sodium in the salt mixture is essential in cardioangiography (Urografin), in which pure sodium or meglumine salts were contraindicated already before the introduction of nonionic CM.

**Synthesis of water-soluble contrast media**
The parent substances for the synthesis of water-soluble CM are iodine and nitrobenzoic acid derivatives. Iodine is a valuable raw material which is obtained partly from marine algae and partly from salt deposits. A significant part of the annual world production of iodine is used for the manufacture of CM.

The complexity of CM synthesis largely depends on the chemical structure of the compound concerned. While ionic CM can be produced from the parent substances in just a few steps, the new nonionic products require a large number of steps (fig. 7). Apart from the expenditure for materials and labor involved in each individual step, some of the material employed – including some of the usually already iodinated precursors – is lost at each step in the synthesis. As an example, even when the yield at each individual step is 90 %, the total yield of an 8-step synthesis is only 43 % of the materials originally employed.

The purification of nonionic CM, which are readily soluble in water, is yet another problem. Ionic CM can be precipitated from water by acid. Nonionic agents cannot be precipitated from water but at most to a limited extent from the customary organic solvents.

Consequently, the extremely high demands made on the quality of CM make the purification of nonionic substances an expensive production step because of the complicated procedures required and the high losses involved.

**The number of steps in CM synthesis**

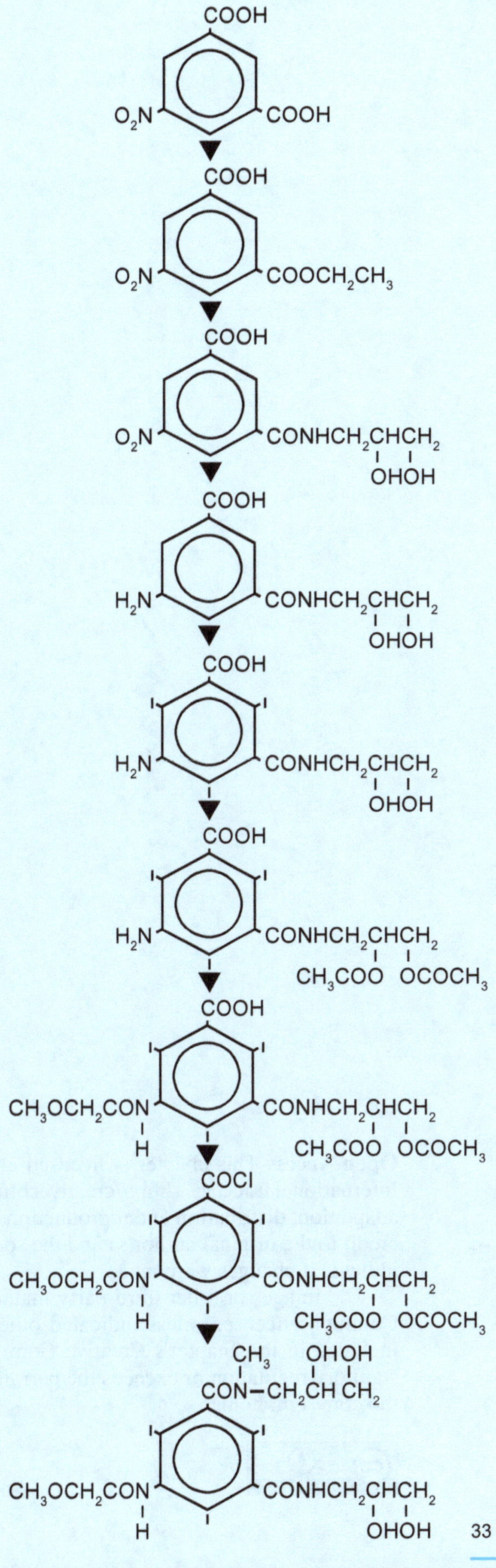

**Fig. 7.** Example of synthesis scheme for water-soluble CM (nonionic)

# DEGRADATION OF IODINATED X-RAY CONTRAST MEDIA

Each year, over 3000 tons of X-ray contrast media are used by medical facilities across the globe. About 90 % of those contrast agents reach our environment largely unaltered through clarification plants. To the present day, degradation products of these substances, which would imply decomposition of the iodinated benzene by microorganisms, have not been identified in sewage sludge.

To estimate possible harmful effects on water and its organisms, toxicological tests with the nonionic iopromide were performed to investigate its effects on water organisms (water flea, two fish species, algae, bacteria) in an environment test system. No toxicological effects on Daphnia magna were observed for short-term (48 hours) exposure to high concentrations of 10 g/l iopromide or long-term exposure (22 days) to lower concentrations of 1 g/l [16].

However, as long as no adequate data on long-term effects of XCM or their synergistic impact on water are available, negative effects cannot be ruled out.


U. Speck, *X-Ray Contrast Media*, https://doi.org/10.1007/978-3-662-56465-3_4

# PHYSICOCHEMICAL PROPERTIES OF WATER-SOLUBLE CONTRAST MEDIA

The most important physicochemical properties of water-soluble, iodinated CM are their solubility, the viscosity and osmolality of the solutions, the lipophilic or hydrophilic properties of the iodine-containing molecule, and the electrical charge (table 4). In practice, these properties have the following significance:

## Water solubility

Very good water solubility is a prerequisite for the production of highly concentrated, radiopaque CM. As with sugars or peptides, the solubility of non-ionic CM is mediated by hydrophilic groups (-OH, -CONH-). Some commercially available CM can crystallize at low temperature and must be dissolved again before use by warming up.

| Property | Significance |
| --- | --- |
| Solubility | Maximum possible concentration; where applicable, need to dissolve crystals in warmth before use |
| Viscosity | Rate of injection; infusion. Highly viscous solutions can impair microcirculation in selective angiography |
| Osmolality | Pain in some angiographic indications; endothelial damage; arachnoiditis(?) in myelography; bradycardia in cardioangiography; hypervolemia after very rapid i.v. injection at high dose; diueresis |
| Lipophilicity, absence of hydrophilia (of ionic CM) | General reactions (nausea, vomiting, allergy-like reactions) more frequent, particularly at high dose and on rapid injection; protein binding, prevention of glomerular filtration; tubular secretion; biliary elimination; permeation through cell membranes, enteral absorption |
| Electric charge | Improvement of solubility; increases the hydrophilia; epileptgenicity |

**Table 4.** The most important physicochemical properties of water-soluble, iodinated CM

© The Author(s) 2018
U. Speck, *X-Ray Contrast Media*, https://doi.org/10.1007/978-3-662-56465-3_5

## Viscosity/Temperature

Viscosity is a measure of the flow properties of a solution and is expressed in millipascal second (identical with the older unit centipoise). It strongly increases with increasing concentration and falling temperature (figs. 8, 9). The viscosity of the different CM is different at the same iodine concentration and same temperature (table 2).

This clearly affects the maximum injection speed, if, e.g., narrow catheters or thin needles are used or if the injection of greater volumes is necessary. Injection speed can be given in mg iodine/ second, as this is the parameter which determines contrast (table 5).

## Osmolality

### Osmotic pressure

The osmotic pressure of a solution can be calculated in two different units, osmolarity and osmolality. The osmolarity is the concentration of osmotically active particles in relation to the volume of a solution. In the case of nonelectrolytes, it is identical to molarity; for dissociated substances $\triangleq$ molarity times the number of ions in one mole; given as osmo/L solution.

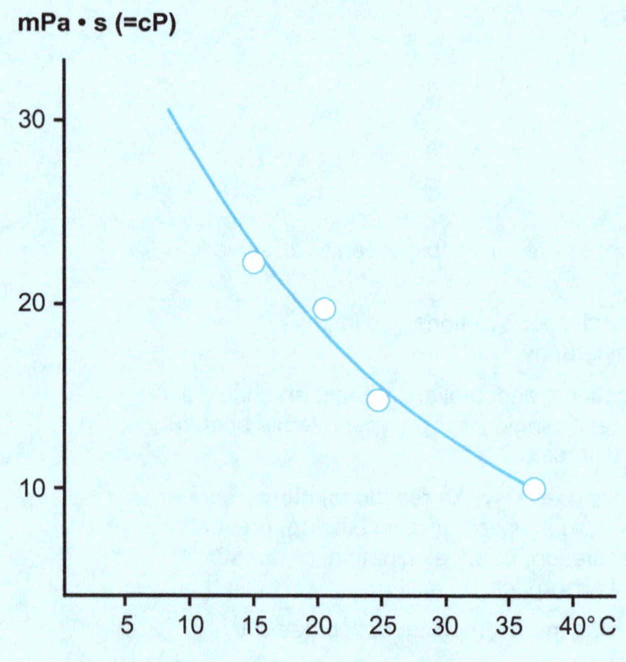


**Fig. 8.** Viscosity of Ultravist in relation to its concentration

**Fig. 9.** Viscosity of Ultravist-370 in relation to temperature

|  | mg Iod/s |
|---|---|
| Ultravist-300 | 2027 |
| Iopamidol-300 | 1974 |
| Ominipaque-300 | 1753 |
| Ominipaque-350 | 1477 |

**Table 5.** Maximum possible injection speed through an 5F headhunter catheter, contrast medium temperature of 37° C; n = 20 per contrast medium [17]

Osmolality describes the concentration of solute per kg of water. The osmolality of CM solutions is expressed in milliosmol/kg water, in megapascal or in atmospheres (1,000 mosm/kg = 2.58 MPa = 25.5 at). It is approximately proportional to the number of freely mobile particles (molecules, ions) per kg water. The osmolality of CM is dependent very much on the concentration and only slightly on the temperature (fig. 10). Different CM can display greatly diverging osmolalities at the same concentration of iodine.

## Hydrophilia/Lipophilia

The lipophilia of iodine-containing CM acids or of nonionic CM is calculated from their distribution between a solvent (octanol, butanol) which is not miscible with water and an aqueous buffer with a pH value (distribution coefficient) close to that of blood or tissues (fig. 11). The electrical charge (acid group) and the oxygen and nitrogen atoms in the side chains reduce the lipophilia of tri-iodobenzene, while methyl groups in the side chains increase it. CM for urography, angiography, CT and myelography should display as little lipophilia as possible.

For ionic contrast media, a correlation was found between lipophilia and certain types of side-effects. This correlation was even more obvious when the degree of binding of the contrast media to plasma proteins was measured rather than lipophilia.

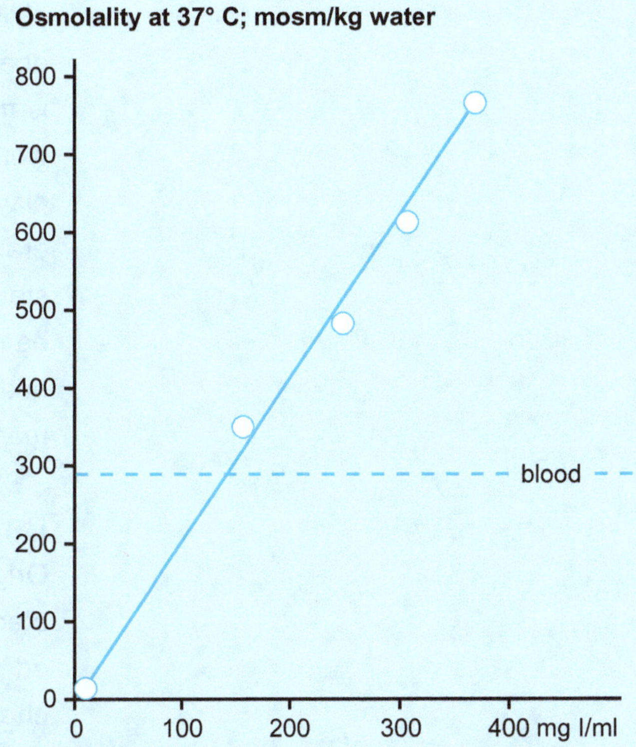


**Fig. 10.** Relationship of the osmolality of Ultravist to the CM concentration

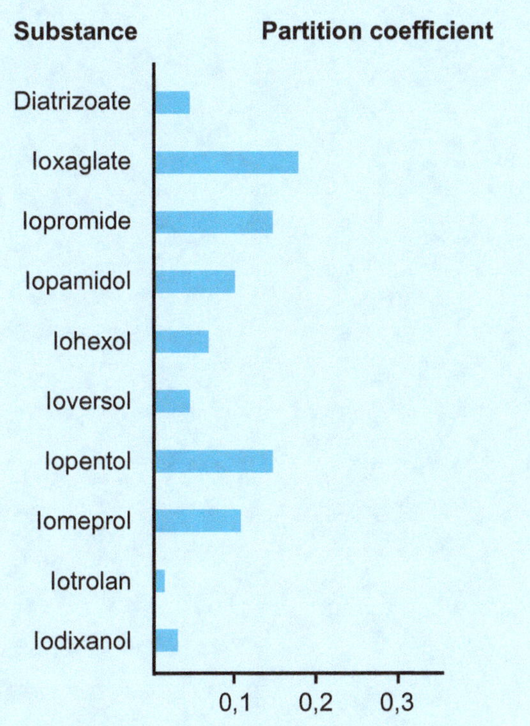


**Fig. 11.** Partition coefficients of different CM between n-butanol and buffer with pH 7.6

Nonionic contrast media are generally very hydrophilic. Their binding to plasma proteins is minor and does not correlate with lipophilia (table 2). The latter is measured as a distribution coefficient (fig. 11). It would seem that hydrogen bonds and other factors play a larger role regarding protein binding and tolerance. Undoubtedly, the tolerance of these substances is also influenced by factors which cannot be measured physicochemically. Cholegraphic CM and particularly the oral ones must be very much more lipophilic to fulfill their purpose.

## Electrical charge

Originally, water-soluble CM were salts of iodinated organic acids. A contrast-producing iodinated anion in solution carries one or two negative charges, whereas a non-contrast-producing cation (e.g., sodium, meglumine) carries one positive electrical charge. Although cations do not directly enhance radiographic imaging, they are essential for improving the solubility of iodinated acids and for attaining physiological pH values. Only acidic CM are effective as biliary contrast media, since only they are eliminated quickly enough by means of a hepatic anion transport mechanism.

For all other indications, the new electrically neutral, nonionic CM have proven more suitable: the cations of CM salts unnecessarily increase the osmolality of the solutions and cause additional, generally undesired effects. The CM ions disturb the electrical potential on cell membranes. Electrical charge is the cause of a host of unwanted interactions of CM with the organism.

## Specific gravity/Density

Concentrated CM solutions are of considerably higher density than water (table 6). The higher density is almost exclusively related to the heavy element iodine. In association with viscosity, the density of CM complicates their miscibility with physiological NaCl solution or blood.

## Others

Several other properties of X-ray contrast media are also of substantial significance. Binding to biomolecules can be mediated not only by the electrical charge and lipophilic groups but also by hydrogen bonds (fig. 12). Hydrogen bonds are responsible for the spatial arrangement of polypeptide chains (folding) and nucleic acids (helix). In many cases they determine the functionality of the macromolecule. The association of X-ray contrast medium molecules with each other in concentrated solution must also be due primarily to hydrogen bonds.

Further relevant properties include the high density (the high specific gravity) of concentrated contrast medium solutions, which hinders the mixing of aqueous solutions with blood, the (minimal) buffering capacity, which ensures rapid assimilation of the contrast medium pH to blood pH, and the powerful absorption of UV light, which is responsible for the light sensitivity of iodinated X-ray contrast media.

|  | mg Iod/ml | Densitiy kg/L 20° C | Densitiy kg/L 37° C |
|---|---|---|---|
| Water |  | 0.998 | 0.993 |
| Ultravist | 150 | 1.154 | 1.158 |
|  | 240 | 1.263 | 1.255 |
|  | 300 | 1.328 |  |
|  | 370 | 1.409 | 1.399 |
| Iopamiron | 200 | 1.223 | 1.216 |
|  | 300 | 1.332 |  |
|  | 370 | 1.415 | 1.405 |
| Omnipaque | 240 | 1.418 | 1.264 |
|  | 300 | 1.343 |  |
|  | 350 | 1.457 | 1.391 |
| Isovist | 240 | 1.285 | 1.269 |
|  | 300 | 1.353 | 1.344 |
| Iopentol | 300 | 1.332 |  |
| Ioversol | 300 | 1.348 |  |
|  | 320 | 1.370 |  |

**Table 6.** Density of different nonionic X-ray contrast agents at 20° and 37°C.

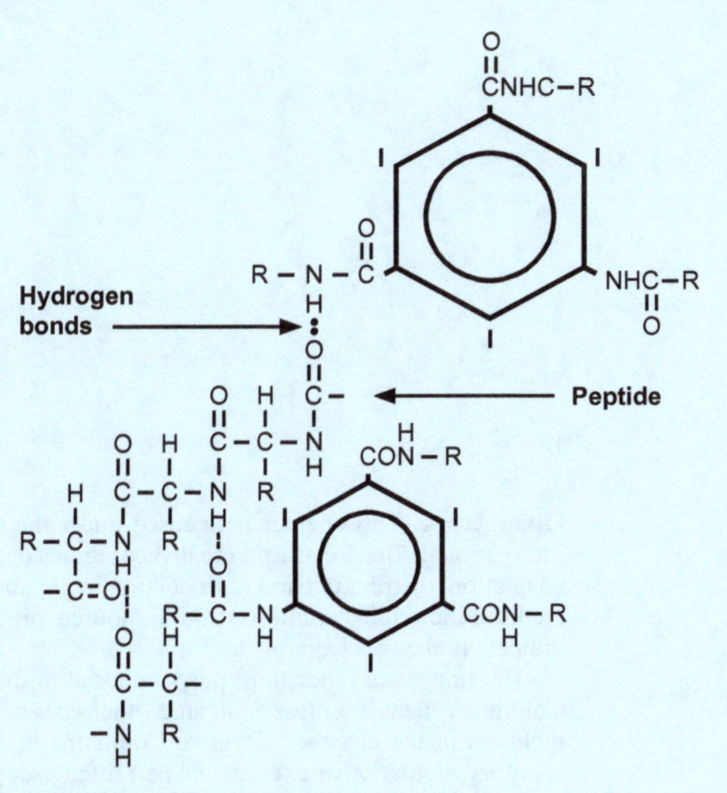

**Fig. 12.** Examples of possible hydrogen bonds (--) between polypeptides and CM

# PHARMACEUTICAL PRODUCT QUALITY

**Practical information at a glance**

| | |
|---|---|
| Proper storage of contrast media | – in a dark place (e.g. in a cupboard)<br>– at room temperatures (15-25° C)<br>– in a warming cabinet at 37° C for no longer than 3 months |
| Observation of expiry dates | – shelf-life of established contrast medium products usually is up to 5 years<br>(as for other pharmaceutical products)<br>– expiry dates displayed on the packaging must be adhered to |
| Examination of the CM solution before use | – remove outer packing only shortly before use<br>– check clearness of solution<br>(no discoloration, no cloudiness, no precipitates) |
| Cystallization found in solution | – can occur at low temperatures (in winter), heat CM solution briefly to 80° C before use; do not use if not completely dissolved |
| CM solution with high viscosity | – heat solution to 37° C, this reduces viscosity and allows solution to drawn up better |
| Risks of microbial contamination | – do not keep opened vials and ampoules longer than one working day after first use; discard all remains at the end of the day |
| Resterilization of the CM solution | – do not resterilize opened containers |
| Transfer into sterile containers | – do not pour CM solution over the unsterile lip of the original container, keep it covered, and do not return it to the original vial |

© The Author(s) 2018

U. Speck, *X-Ray Contrast Media*, https://doi.org/10.1007/978-3-662-56465-3_6

## Purity of the active ingredient, by-products and degradation products

Because of the high doses employed - which can exceed 100 g of substance per patient and examination – very high demands are made on CM in terms of chemical purity. The molecular structure of the CM substance is confirmed by NMR (nuclear magnetic resonance), , IR (infra red), MS (mass spectrometry) and UV (ultraviolet) spectra (fig. 13a-e).

In addition, contrast media are tested for foreign substances using thin-layer chromatography (fig. 13e) and high-pressure liquid chromatography (HPLC) to identify any by-products originating from synthesis [18, 19]. The total iodine content is calculated by means of micro-iodine determination following wet combustion of a sample; the active ingredient content is determined by spectral photometric measurement or HPLC.

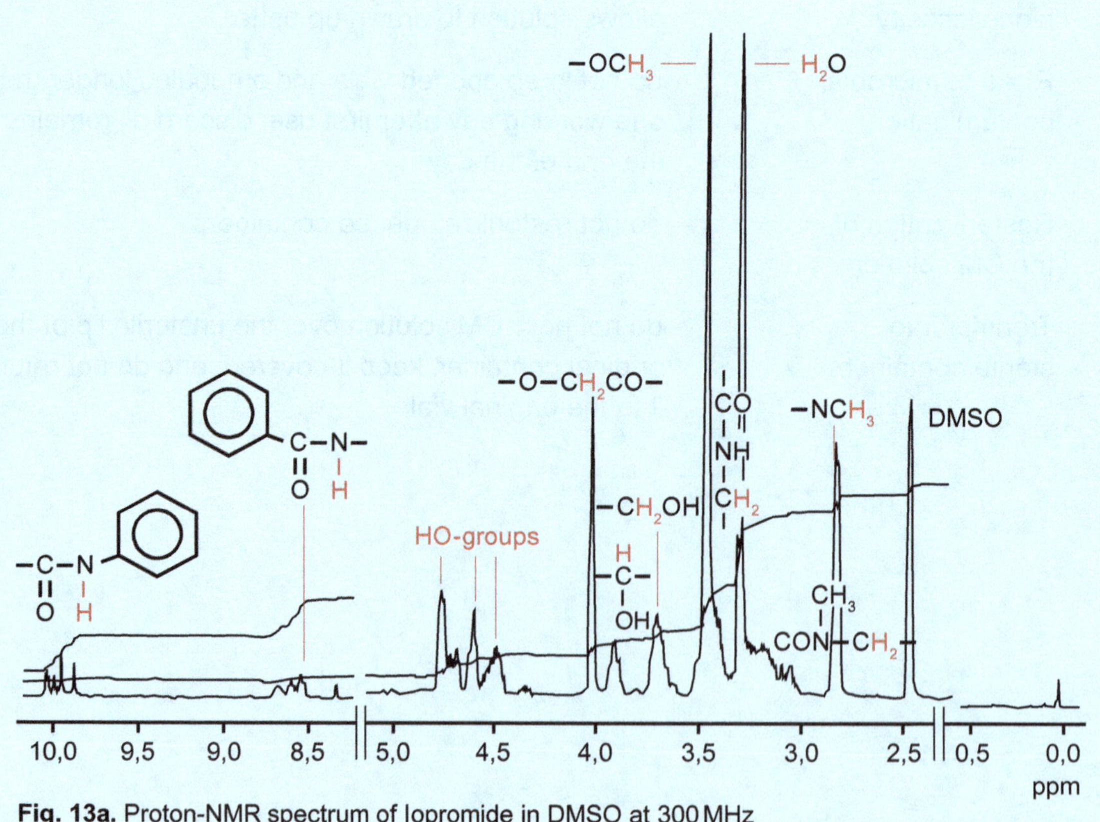


**Fig. 13a.** Proton-NMR spectrum of Iopromide in DMSO at 300 MHz

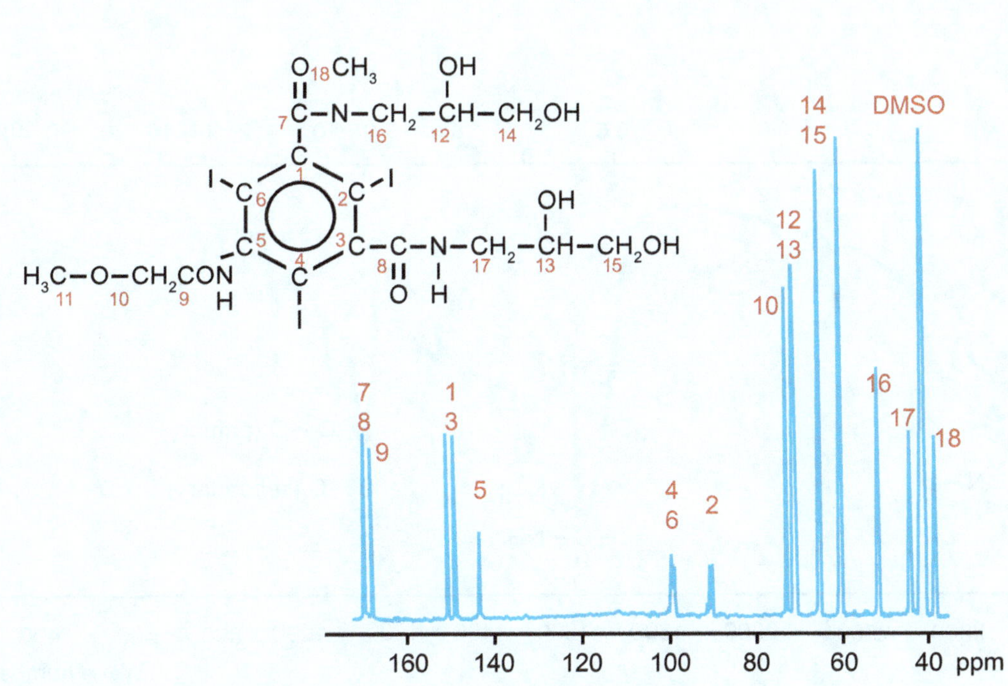

**Fig. 13b.** ¹³C-NMR-spectrum of Iopromide in DMSO at 75.5 MHz

The prescribed values for CM content are 98-102 %. In addition, tests for purity are performed using suitable customary pharmacopoeia methods: these include evaluation of color, clarity and pH of the test solution; water content, sulfate ash, and heavy metal contamination and tests for anorganic iodide and aromatic amine; TLC (thin-layer chromatography) for foreign substances. Nonionic CM are also tested for ionic contamination by measuring their conductivity.

Two particular reactions are of importance with regard to the storage of CM solutions: hydrolysis of amide bonds and cleavage of iodide [20].

Hydrolysis is suggested either by (additional) free carboxyl groups occurring at the aromate (with a strongly acidic reaction) and aliphatic amines or by the occurrence of aliphatic carbonic acids and aromatic amines.

Cleavage of iodine from the aromate leads to an increase of iodide in the solution; no elementary iodine is released. Degradation reactions of CM usually manifest as changes in pH.

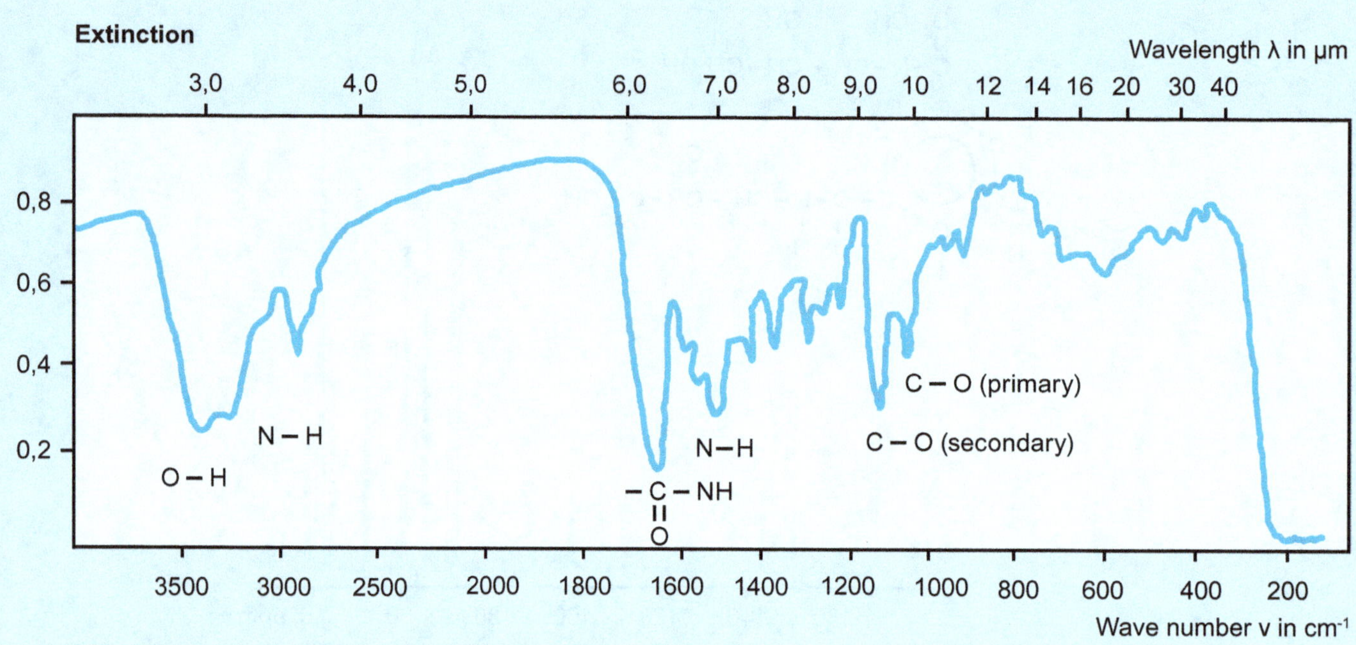


**Fig. 13c.** Infrared spectrum of Iopromide in KBr

## Formulations

X-ray contrast media are usually offered as ready-to-inject aqueous solutions with the exception of Lipiodol and barium sulphate. Attention must be paid to the following properties with regard to use:

- type and amount of the CM substance,
- where applicable, type or mixture of salts,
- iodine concentration in the solution in mg/ml.

However, it has to be kept in mind that the concentration of the active ingredient in the CM solution alone rarely allows predicting opacification.

## Additives

In addition to the CM substance and water, the finished preparations also contain pharmacologically relevant adjuvants. $CaNa_2EDTA$ (calcium disodium ethylene-diamine tetraacetic acid) is pharmacologically virtually inactive in the concentrations used. It is employed as a stabilizer to prevent iodide release from the organic bond caused by heavy metal catalysis, e.g., by traces of $Cu^{2+}$. Sodium EDTA used to be added for this purpose, but its calcium-binding property led to a reduction of cardiac contractility in cardio-angiography.

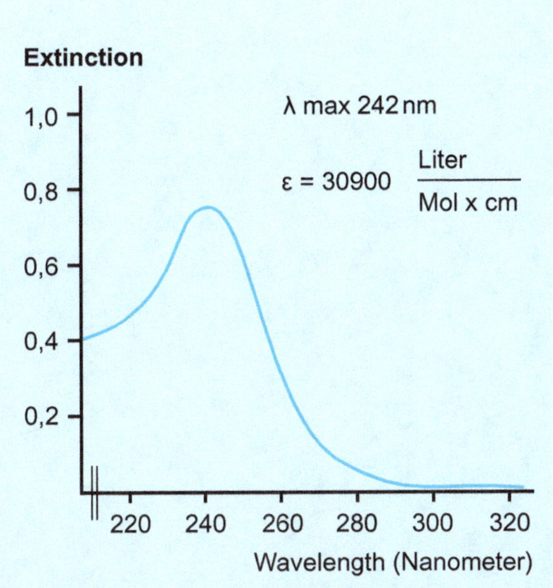



**Fig. 13d.** Ultraviolet spectrum of iopromide in water (24 µg iopromide/ml slice thickness = 1 cm)

**Fig. 13e.** Thin-layer chromatogram of iopromide on a silica gel plate 60F-254 (Merck). Solvent: dioxane (85)-water (15)-ammonia (4). Amounts applied from left to right: 200 µg, 100 µg, 50 µg, 1 µg, 50 µg, 100 µg, 200 µg. Photograph taken at 254 nm

This effect is not observed with $CaNa_2EDTA$ [21]. Formulations of the nonionic CM Ultravist and Omnipaque contain 0.1 mg/ml $CaNa_2EDTA$.

Buffers can be added to stabilize the pH of CM during storage. Tris and carbonate buffers, of which only low concentrations are required, are particularly suitable. The pH of CM solutions is approximately in the physiological range. The buffering effect is only slight.

After injection, the pH quickly adapts to that of blood. The formulations of Omnipaque and Ultravist contain 1.21 and 2.42 mg/ml Tris, respectively, with chloride as the counterion.

Preservatives (parabenes) may be present in CM for retrograde urography, while oral CM for examinations of the GI tract may contain flavoring agents and emulsifiers.

## Microbiological quality of the finished product

### Production under controlled environmental conditions

The manufacture of solutions for injection and infusion requires special hygienic measures determined by the production facilities, the technical equipment and the workers' competence.

Manufacturers must meet not only international and national legal regulations and guidelines for pharmaceutical products, but also the much stricter requirements for the production of X-ray contrast media (fig. 14 a-f).

Further reduction of microbiological contamination is achieved by dividing the entire working area into cleanliness classes:

Designing production rooms as differently controlled areas aims at preventing possible particular and microbiological impurities and cross-contaminations while producing contrast media:

**CRCA:** Clean room Class A – rooms for hazardous work processes (aseptic production and filling, irrelevant for production of final sterilized products)

**CRCB:** Clean room Class B – surrounding area of CRCA in case of aseptic production and filling

**CRCC:** Clean room Class C – Filling of solutions without extraordinary risk of particulate matter and microbiological contamination

**CRCD:** Clean room Class D – production of bulk-solutions without extraordinary risk for microbiological and particulate matter contamination

An air-conditioning system regulated centrally via microprocessor provides for the necessary environmental conditions at the individual workplaces. In aseptic working zones, laminar-flow units - special filter units – in addition to the conventional sterile air supply protect the product from the risk of contamination by man and environment.

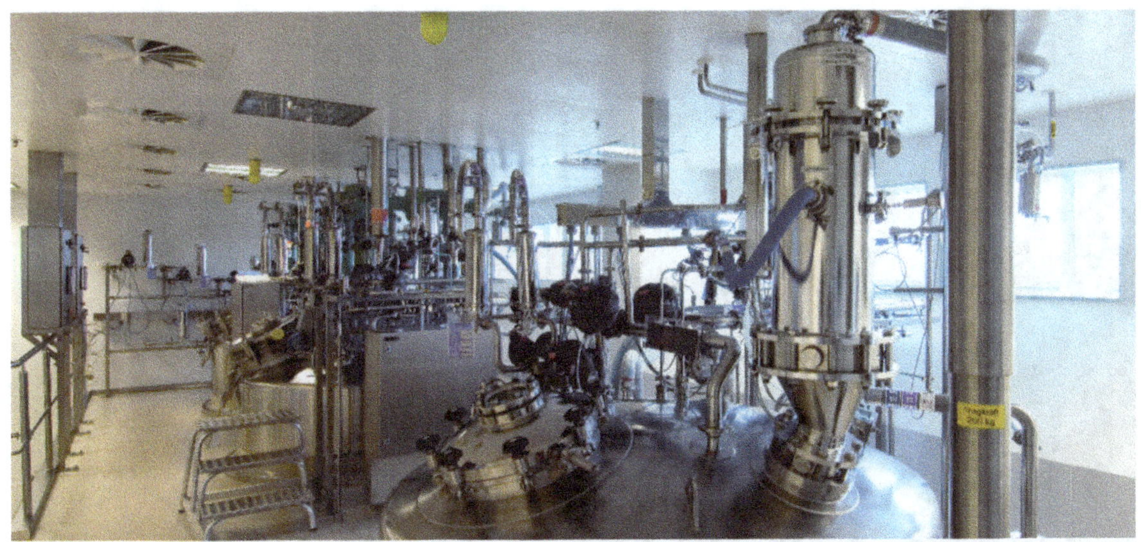

**Fig. 14a.** Production of solutions and temporary storage

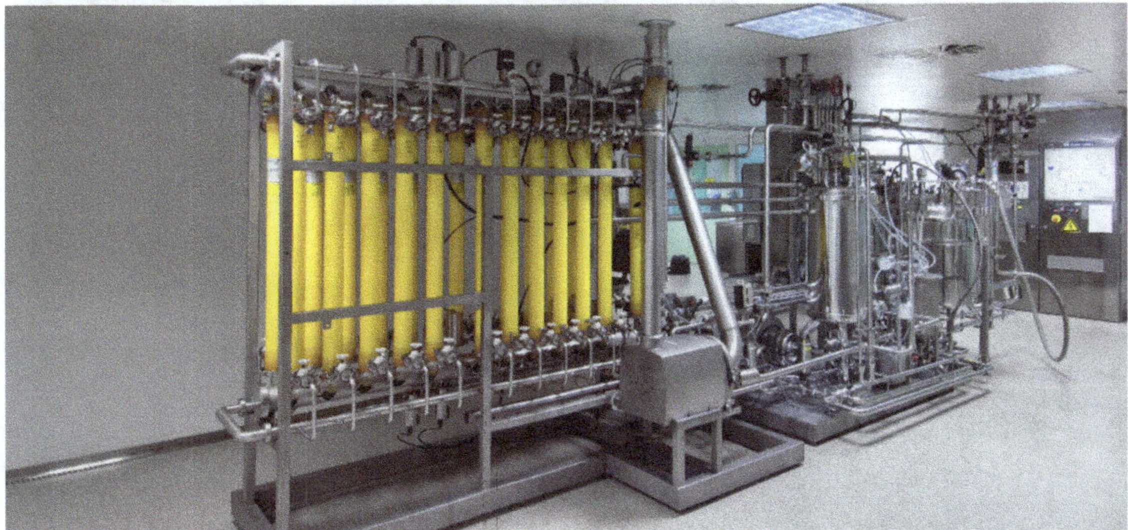

**Fig. 14b.** Ultrafiltration facility

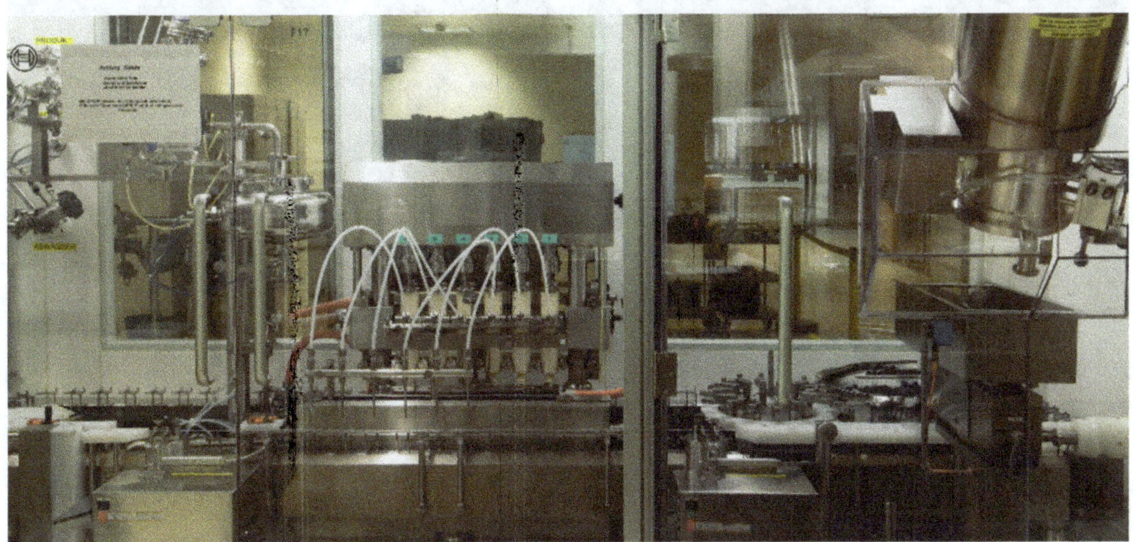

**Fig. 14c.** Infusion bottle line - filling machine under laminar flow

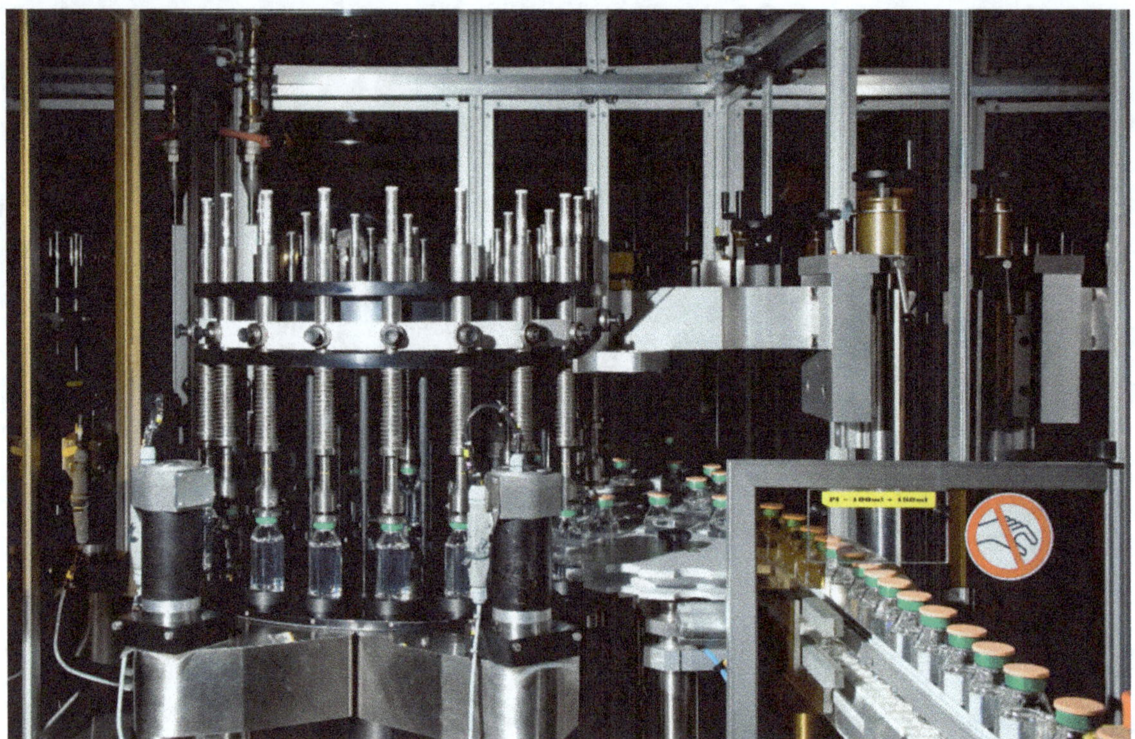

**Fig. 14d.** Electronic control of infusion bottles

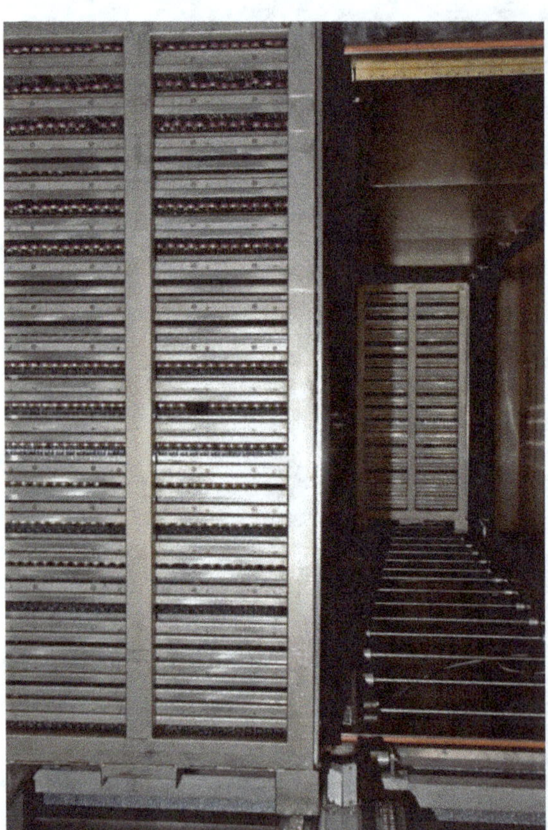

**Fig. 14e.** Sterilisation

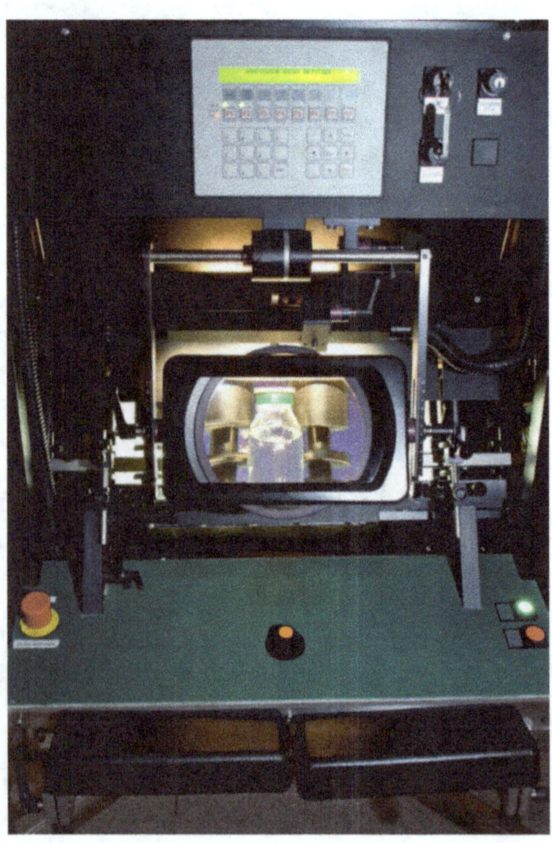

**Fig. 14f.** Visual control of infusion bottles

Mechanical production lines have been automated as much as possible to reduce the risks which can arise through direct contact between staff and products during these procedural steps. Examples are computer-controlled cleaning processes for cleaning agitators, pressure tanks and other equipment.

Strict observance of all pharmaceutical rules and the proper use of technical equipment require qualified staff consisting of pharmacists, engineers, technicians and skilled workers, who undergo regular training and thus apply the latest scientific and technical insights.

**Production process**
Table 7 provides a simplified schematic production flow of CM manufacture.

Of interest here is the number of steps in the production. Each production step is followed by a process control step to ensure that a given production step has been carried out as specified before the next step is initiated . Thus, the sum of the results of the individual process control steps describes the quality of the finished product and says more about it than the finished article or final control, the result of which can only be based on selected samples.

Let's just follow the production flow described in table 7:
The ingredients and packing material are checked as they come in and, after release by quality control and cleaning of the outer surfaces, are packed on pallets for intermediate storage.

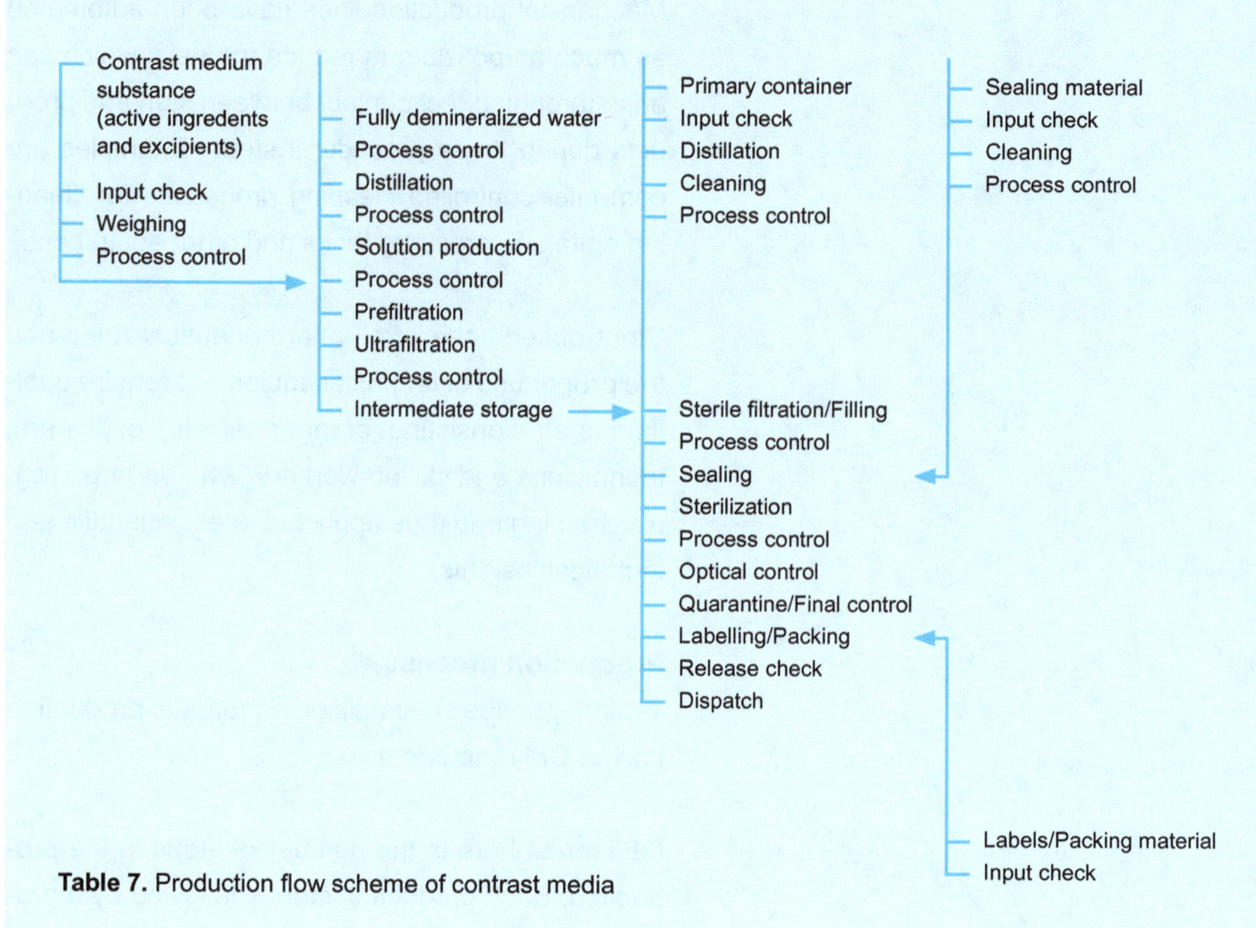


**Table 7.** Production flow scheme of contrast media

The amounts of active substance and adjuvants specified in the prescription for a batch of the respective preparation are weighed in a weighing center and the data documented via an automatic control system. After an identity check, the substances are brought in special containers to the make-up rooms and dissolved in a stirring apparatus.

The various chemical and physical data of the testing standard are checked before the solution undergoes sterile filtration. During filtration, all micro-organisms and contaminating particles are sieved out of the solution. Particles down to a size of a 5,000th of a millimeter can be filtered out. After this step, the solutions are ready for filling and are led into the filling plant via a special system of pipes.

Vials are cleaned, for instance by ultrasound, sterilized, filled and sealed in a special cleaning, filling and sealing machine. The process is accompanied by a check on the amount filled.

Although the fact that the production rooms are aseptic means that filling can take place without contamination from the environment, the filling machines are further protected by a laminar-flow arrangement. The filled and sealed containers undergo final sterilization in steam autoclaves.

Finally, all filled products are examined for possible particulate contamination.

Optical inspection can be done fully automatically or visually. Visual inspection is performed by specifically educated staff. During the inspection, the objects rotate in front of an illuminated background and are observed through a magnifier. Different options exist for fully automatic inspection:
- Measurement of attenuation of light intensity caused by particles using an Evaporative Light Scattering Detector (ELSD)
- Evaluation of photographs of the rotating probes
- A combination of the above

The final medical product batch is then transferred to a quarantine storage house and approved for packaging after a final control by the pharmaceutical quality management.

**Sterile filtration, ultrafiltration and sterilization**
All starting materials, such as active ingredients, pure water, containers and stoppers, are constantly checked for microbial contaminations.

Sterile filtration of the solutions and sterilization of the filled containers ensure the necessary sterility. In addition, what is known as molecular or ultrafiltration can be performed. This process is used in the production of contrast media like Ultravist and is able to retain molecules above a molecular weight of 10,000 D. It ensures that not only micro-organisms but also their high-molecular-weight metabolic products including pyrogens are withdrawn, resulting in a distinct reduction of the particle content in the lower micrometer range. In addition, the CM solution passes through a sterile filter while it is being filled into the vials.

Finally, the finished, firmly sealed individual containers are autoclaved for 20 min at 121° C. The containers are heated for the shortest possible time by superheated steam and cooled again quickly by being sprayed with water. This is important because the chemical stability of the CM is limited at such high temperatures.

## Sterility test

Sterility testing is done to check whether micro-organisms capable of multiplication can be demonstrated in the final product. Sterility is tested using the Millipore-Steritest system for two culture media. The contents of 20 containers from each batch manufactured in the production line undergo membrane filtration via the Steritest system: the membrane, which has an average pore diameter of $\leq 0.45\,\mu m$, retains any micro-organisms present.

The contents of each container are distributed evenly to two filter units and filtered. One filter is then coated with the culture medium casein-peptone/soyapeptone bouillon, the other filter with thioglycolate medium. The entire filter units are incubated for 10 days to allow micro-organisms to grow. At the end of the incubated period, the filter units are checked for macroscopically visible growth (turbidity). The sterility requirements are fulfilled when the culture media remain clear after brief shaking.

## Test for pyrogens

Fever reactions can occur in humans and animals after parenteral administration of injection and infusion solutions. The reactions are frequently caused by microbial metabolic and degradation products or endotoxins (constituents of the cell walls of gram-negative bacteria). These fever-producing substances with a chemically heterogeneous structure are known as pyrogens.

The commonest internationally used test to detect and quantitate endotoxic contamination by gram-negative bacteria in drugs is the LAL (limulus amebocyte lysate) test, which is described in detail in the relevant pharmacopoeias. It is named after the horseshoe crab Limulus polyphemus, because the amebocyte lysate of its blood is used in the test.

Different techniques can be used to perform the LAL test:
• Gel-clot method (based on gel formation)
• Turbidimetric method (based on turbidity after cleavage of an endogeneous substrate)
• Chromogenic method (based on colour formation after cleavage of peptide chromogen complex)

The LAL test, an in vitro pyrogen test, is a limited alternative to the rabbit test, which is an in vivo pyrogen test to detect pyrogenic contamination in drugs.

Rabbits react quickly to the slightest pyrogenic impurity in an intravenously injected solution with an increase of body temperature. The method of testing is described in detail in the relevant pharmacopoeias. Although the rabbit test is not mandatory in Europe and the US anymore, it is still used in some countries. The LAL test is limited by the fact that it is only able to specifically demonstrate bacterial endotoxins. The latter are the most common impurities with the highest pyrogenic activity.

After filling and sterilization, the CM undergo a final
and thorough quality check. After manufacture, it
may be a while before the products are actually
used – a period in which the products are transport-
ed and stored under varying conditions. Finally, the
vials are opened or the stoppers are pierced, and
the CM solution is drawn up directly into syringes
or automatic injectors. It may be infused through
an infusion kit or transferred to another container.
The content of a vial is to be used up immediately
after opening.

Transport, storage and handling during use may
impair the quality of a CM solution. A number of
influences to which the products may be exposed
after the final control by the manufacturer have
been simulated in the laboratory and examined for
their effect on the quality of the solutions. The user
should always recheck the clarity of the solution
immediately before use (see page 38).

**Stability in long-term storage and at different
temperatures**

One of the most important checks on CM solutions concerns their long-term stability. To ensure
high quality up to actual use, every effort is made
to develop the CM formulation and to choose the
container materials in such a way that storage under normal conditions is possible for up to 5 years.
Since insufficient experience is usually available
at the time a new product is introduced to be able
to prove such sustained stability; an expiry date
on the order of 2 or 3 years is usually stated as a
precaution.

The stability of CM is satisfactory at room temperature (15-25° C); there is no need to store the products in a cool place unless this is expressly mentioned on the label. Ionic CM (Gastrografin, etc.) can crystallize at temperatures close to freezing point, e.g., during transport in winter.

The crystals are usually easily recognizable and can be dissolved again in the unopened vial by brief heating to a maximum of 80° C. Contrast media generally tolerate such brief heating without any problems, since they are heated to 121° C for 20 min after manufacture for final sterilization. The same naturally applies to warming the solution to body temperature before use to improve tolerance. Renewed sterilization of solutions from opened containers is not permitted.

Although prolonged storage (for months or years) at higher temperatures (e.g., 30° C) does not result in surpassing the limits of the product's quality specifications, it should be avoided because higher temperatures accelerate degradation reactions.

Appearance alone does not always allow the user to recognize CM which no longer meet the quality specifications. Typical analytical changes are a decreased pH and an increase of iodide and degradation products. Discoloration, turbidity and sedimentation can be recognized with the naked eye and indicate imperfect quality.

| pH value | 6.5–8.0 |
|---|---|
| Free amine | ≤0.1% |
| Iodide | ≤75 µg/ml solution |
| Color | ≤ color of comparison solution B5 or BG5 or G5 |
| Content of active ingredient | ≤95–105% |

**Table 8.** Quality features and their threshold values with Ultravist-240 as the example

When stored correctly, i.e., protected from light and X-rays, and when observing the limits for storage temperature and duration, the critical values listed in table 8 will not be exceeded. Ultravist-240, Ultravist-300, and Ultravist-370 are still stable even after storage for several years at temperatures of both 20°C and 30°C (table 9).

**Sensitivity to irradiation and light: white glass, brown glass, and UV-protective foil**

X-ray contrast media are sensitive to light and, to some extent, also to irradiation. They should be stored in the dark and for only a limited time close to X-ray units.

Although brown glass or UV-protective foil provides some protection against light, it has the major disadvantage that any particles which may occur (fragments of the stopper, crystals) are less easy to recognize. It is for this important reason that containers made of colorless glass are preferred.

| | Storage period | Iodide (µg/ml) | | pH value | | Substance content as % | |
|---|---|---|---|---|---|---|---|
| | | 20° C | 30° C | 20° C | 30° C | 20° C | 30° C |
| Ultravist-240 | 0 | 1 | | 7.62 | | 100 | |
| 50 ml | 24 months | 6 | 11 | 7.51 | 7.50 | 99 | 99 |
| Ultravist-300 | 0 | 3 | | 7.52 | | 100 | |
| 50 ml | 24 months | 6 | 14 | 7.34 | 7.23 | 99 | 100 |
| Ultravist-370 | 0 | 3 | | 7.30 | | 100 | |
| 50 ml | 24 months | 13 | 35 | 7.29 | 7.09 | 99 | 99 |

**Table 9.** Stability data of different formulations/ strengths of a nonionic CM

Because usually the glass is colorless, however, it is especially important that the outer packing (carton etc.) not be removed until shortly before use or that the CM be stored in a dark place, e.g., in a cupboard. During normal manipulation and use, exposure to light of normal room brightness (approx. 600 lux, cf. fig. 15) is not critical, but exposure to sunlight must be avoided.

The sensitivity to X-ray irradiation is quite low. Irradiation of up to 10 rd produced no relevant effect on either Urografin or Ultravist (table 10).

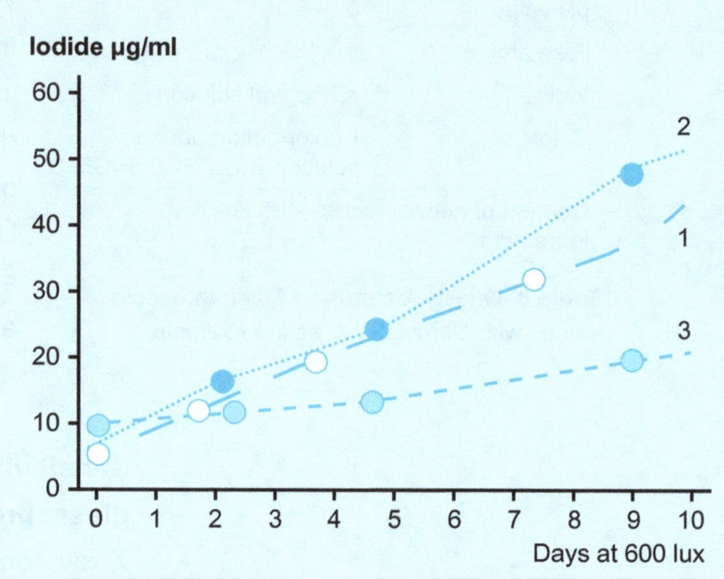


**Fig. 15.** Release of Iodide from 3 different CM stored in a 50-ml clear glass vial and illuminated

| | Description<br>Color | pH<br>value | Iodide<br>(µg/ml) | Free amine<br>(%) |
|---|---|---|---|---|
| **Urografin 30 %**<br>Nonirradiated | clear, colorless solution;<br>< G6 | 6.63 | 3.7 | 0.006 |
| **Urografin 30 %**<br>1 rd irradiated | Unchanged | 6.62 | 3.6 | 0.004 |
| **Urografin 30 %**<br>10 rd irradiated | Unchanged | 6.62 | 3.6 | 0.006 |
| **Ultravist-300**<br>Nonirradiated | clear, colorless solution;<br>G6 | 7.60 | 2.5 | 0.017 |
| **Ultravist-300**<br>1 rd irradiated | Unchanged | 7.60 | 3.2 | 0.017 |
| **Ultravist-300**<br>10 rd irradiated | Unchanged | 7.60 | 3.3 | 0.018 |

**Table 10.** Effects of X-ray irradiation on CM solution

**Tests for contamination with particles**

Particles in the X-ray CM solution must be avoided at all costs. They represent one of the most serious problems in the manufacture and handling because X-ray CM – unlike most infusion solutions – are injected not only intravenously but sometimes intra-arterially into the vessels of highly sensitive organs [22]. After their production, CM are checked very carefully for their content of the most minute particles. Particles subsequently occurring in closed containers may be CM crystals, which appear in individual solutions when kept at temperatures close to or below the freezing point. Unopened vials containing noncrystalline flocculation and unopened nonionic CM vials containing crystals or sediments are to be returned to the manufacturer immediately. Crystals – when caused by storage at low temperature – can be dissolved again as described on page 38.

Contamination with particles can occur upon removal of the CM from the original container [23]. One possible cause is fragmentation of the stopper material. The punching-out of rubber particles and the formation of rubber shavings cannot be fully avoided when a rubber stopper is pierced by a cannula. This also applies, of course, to the sticker of infusion kits, although the kits offered by some manufacturers are fitted with appropriate fluid filters.

For testing purposes, stoppers were fitted to normal vials and pierced with cannulas. After a total of 20 stoppers were each pierced 5 times, i.e., after 100 piercings, the fragments are washed off, isolated on membrane filters and then counted.

Comparative studies show that fragmentation is essentially dependent on the quality of cannula sharpening and cannula caliber.

Other factors with a less marked effect on fragmentation include stopper geometry, especially the thickness of the membrane that is pierced, and the stopper elastomer, its content of filler and hardness.

Handling also has a considerable influence. For example, care must be taken to never insert the cannula in exactly the same place twice when multiple doses are removed. Since most CM are offered as so-called single-dose preparations, however, this risk is avoided.

Even the shape in which the cannula is ground is important. Only cannulas ground to an acute or moderately acute angle should be used for piercing stoppers. Cannulas ground at an obtuse angle, e.g., those used as indwelling venous cannulas, increase the rate of fragmentation considerably. It goes without saying that the ground surface must be perfect. Cannulas which have become blunted, e.g., because they have been used several times and have hit the bottom of the vial, should be discarded.

The fragmentation rate obviously increases with the caliber of the cannula. Fragmentation of the stoppers increases decisively between 16G and 18G cannulas.

There is a temptation to use a larger cannula to shorten the time taken to draw up the solution, particularly when, for example, 50 ml of a relatively viscous CM solution is required. Instead, it is possible to reduce viscosity by about a half by warming the solution to 37° C. Moreover, so-called combi stoppers need not be pierced and, instead, can be removed after tearing off the flanged cap. Of course, the solution can then only be drawn up with a syringe or with the syringe of a high-pressure injector. In the interest of sterility, the solution should not be poured out over the lip of the vial.

Finally, there is also a possibility of particle contamination from syringes and catheters, and this is likewise very difficult to detect.

## Risks of microbial contamination

Tri-iodinated CM were originally developed from antibacterial substances. The ionic CM still on the market have distinct antimicrobial activity, at least in the customary high concentrations of 300 mg I/ml or more. This effect is attributable to two factors:

- the high osmolality and
- a residue of chemotoxicity.

In contrast, nonionic CM are a good culture medium for fungi and bacteria because of their chemical composition and tolerance [24].

The behavior of micro-organisms in a nonionic CM solution was studied in various Ultravist solutions (fig. 16). Six specimens of different groups of micro-organism were used as representatives of a broad spectrum of pathogens.

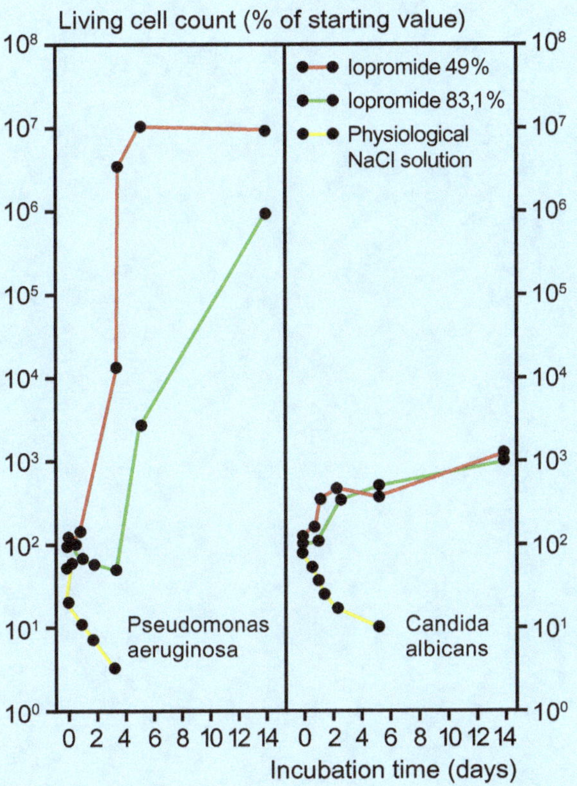



**Fig. 16.** Development of Candida albicans and Pseudomonas aeruginosa in aqueous solutions of a nonionic CM (Ultravist) at room temperature over a period of 14 days (incubation time)

The risk of microbial multiplication and spoiling of the product were simulated by artificial contamination in a model experiment:

Three of the 6 types of micro-organisms grew in Ultravist solutions:

- Pseudomonas aeruginosa (gram-negative bacterium, rod-shaped bacillus)
- Candida albicans (fungus, yeast)
- Aspergillus niger (fungus, mold).

The growth of Staphylococcus aureus (gram-positive bacterium, coccus) was inhibited. The Ultravist solution had no effects on gram-positive, sporiferous bacteria: Bacillus subtilis (aerobic) and Clostridium sporogenes (anaerobic). Neither an increase nor a decrease of the germ count was found for these organisms.

The risk of microbial contamination of the CM in the production zone can be kept low if, during the manufacture, filling and sterilization, the time between making up the solution and subsequent antimicrobial treatment is kept as short as possible.

The following advice applies to the use of nonionic CM in particular:

- Careful avoidance of contamination of solutions and materials which come into contact with the solutions.
- Opened vials and ampoules to be used up in the course of one examination session if possible; keep for no longer than one working day after opening or removal of the first dose.
- All remains to be discarded at the end of a day to prevent their subsequent use.

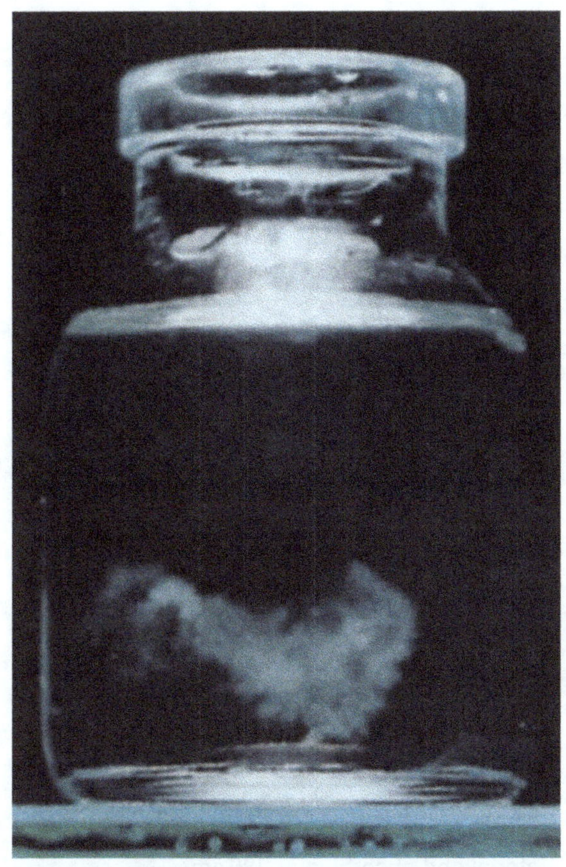

**Fig. 17.** Example of a microbially contaminated contrast medium solution. About 10 yeast cells were injected through the rubber stopper into the previously sterile contrast medium vial and then kept for about 3 weeks at room temperature. The development and maintenance of a fungal mycelium are promoted by the viscosity of the solution

Microbial contamination of CM solutions can, of course, only be recognized macroscopically at a very late stage. Fungal infection is characterized by a cloud of suspended particles resembling a cotton swab (fig. 17).

### Transferring the contrast medium to sterile containers, disposable syringes, automatic injectors

Apart from the primary container, CM almost invariably come into contact with other containers, with syringes, tubes, catheters, injection needles, etc.

### Transferring to sterile containers

Some X-ray examinations must be performed under absolutely aseptic conditions. In these cases, the CM is transferred to, for example, sterile containers, since the unsterile outer surface of the original container would be a possible source of contamination. Measures to be followed here are:

- The CM solution should not be poured over the unsterile lip of the original container, but should be removed with a large-caliber cannula after complete removal of the stopper.
- The solution should be covered to prevent drying-out with crystal formation.
- Stability in an open container is, of course, limited to a short time; under no circumstances should solutions be returned to the original vial.

**Drawing-up into disposable syringes or automatic injectors**

When CM solutions are being drawn up from the original container into disposable syringes or filled into the syringes of high-pressure injectors, there exists − as with all opened vials − the risk of microbial contamination and subsequent multiplication as well as the possibility that ingredients of the plastic material or plunger will diffuse into the CM solution [25]. In all cases, the CM should not be drawn up into the syringes until immediately before use.

Table 11 shows a particularly unfavorable example. Constituents able to diffuse have been identified as 2-mercaptobenzothiazole and 2-hydroxyethylmer cabo benzothiazole. They reach concentrations of up to several µg/ml.

| Hours | $E_{280\,nm}$ | pH |
|---|---|---|
| 0 | 0 | 6.8 |
| 1 | 0.05 | 6.7 |
| 2 | 0.10 | 6.3 |
| 4 | 0.16 | 6.6 |
| 7.5 | 0.29 | 6.2 |
| 22 | 0.57 | 6.3 |
| 24 | 0.58 | 6.4 |

**Table 11.** Alteration of an unbuffered aqueous solution in a disposable syringe caused by substances entering the solution from the syringe material and absorbing at 280 nm

**Use of large-volume CM bottles**

For intravascular CM investigations, large-volume bottles (500 ml) are sometimes used for reasons of economy, easier handling and better radiation protection of staff. The contrast media are administered with automatic injectors or infusion pumps, which are filled from the 500 ml bottles using appropriate transfer systems. Intentionally unfavorable conditions such as touching the surface of the stopper or the mini-spike with the fingers were created in carefully designed studies but even these conditions caused only minimal contamination of the contrast media. No proliferation of micro-organisms in Ultravist was observed within 24 hours [26, 27]. Likewise, under the conditions of angiography, no relevant microbial contamination had appeared by the end of the angiographic examination when Ultravist was left in open containers [27].

# PHARMACOLOGICAL PROPERTIES OF CM

### Biochemical-pharmacological properties

Contrast agents influence the human organism not only because of their physical properties such as osmolality, viscosity and hydrophilicity but also because of their special chemical structure. Contrary to former beliefs, effects are not induced by free iodine, but by the contrast medium molecule. Hemodynamic, neurological and pseudoallergic effects are partially attributable to the chemical structure of contrast media molecules.

Several biochemical reactions are more or less related to the general tolerance of XCM.

### Protein binding

Contrast agents show variable binding to albumin in blood plasma after intravascular administration. Albumin binding is strongly enhanced by a free/ unsubstituted position five of the benzene ring, which is intentionally the case in intravenous cholegraphics. Those substances show an albumin binding of up to 90 % [28].

All uroangiographic contrast agents in use today are substituted in position five of the benzene ring and possess additional hydroxyl groups (-OH) and other hydrophilic groups (-CON), which make protein binding practically impossible.

© The Author(s) 2018
U. Speck, *X-Ray Contrast Media*, https://doi.org/10.1007/978-3-662-56465-3_7

The following percentages of plasma protein binding were found in a large comparative study: 14 % for the ionic dimeric ioxaglinic acid, 8.8 % for the ionic diatrizoic acid, and 4.3 % and 1.8 % for the dimeric nonionic contrast agents iodixanol and iotrolan. The nonionic iopromide showed an extremely low binding of < 1 % [29].

## Complement activation

Many clinical observations and experimental studies showed XCM to be able to activate factors of the complement system, the kinin system, other mediators, and eventually the blood coagulation system as well as the fibrinolytic system.

A radioimmunoassay (RIA) study shows that different ionic and nonionic contrast agents may in vitro activate fraction C3 of the complement system and additionally release anaphylatoxin C3a and C5a [30].

The exact mechanism of complement activation is still debated. However, it appears to occur without involvement of Ig-complexes via the alternative pathway [31].

## Enzyme inhibition

Plasma enzymes such as ß- glucoronidase, lysozyme, alcohol dehydrogenase and glucose-6-phosphate dehydrogenase are unspecifically inhibited by binding with CM, without this inhibition being clinically relevant.

Conversely, inhibition of plasma acetycholinesterase by CM may contribute to pseudoallergic reactions such as urticaria, gastrointestinal symptoms and vasodilatation.

A comparison of iopromide and iopamidol at concentrations of 0 to 40 mgI/ml showed the inhibition of acetylcholinesterase to be dose-dependent with 15% inhibition at the highest concentration of both CM [32].

Angiotensin-converting enzyme (ACE) is equally strongly inhibited by ionic and nonionic XCM in in-vitro studies. Inhibition is determined by the chelates used as stabilizers in the contrast agents.

ACE of the pulmonary vascular endothelial surface inactivates bradykinin entirely through hydrolytic degradation during lung passage. Bradykinin is closely associated with anaphylactoid reactions to contrast agents [33].

## Influence on blood cells

The influence of XCM on red and white blood cells, on thrombocytes and the blood coagulation system is complex and not yet fully understood. In vivo and in vitro studies often show divergent results.

Red blood cells

XCM cause variable, concentration-dependent osmotic shrinkage of erythrocytes, which is related to physicochemical features of the substance and also to its chemical toxicity. Due to the osmotic effect of the hypertonic blood-CM mixture, potassium and liquid pass from erythrocytes into the plasma. Metrizamide or iodipamide solutions of low osmolality modify the membrane  of erythrocytes in such a way that they assume a spiky shape (echinocytes) [34, 35].

This transformation reduces the blood cell's elasticity and thus affects blood flow velocity through small capillaries. This effect is rarely observed after injection of nonionic XCM.

White blood cells

After injection of iopromide and the dimeric ionic ioxaglate, the number of leukocytes dropped in patients who underwent arteriography. Nevertheless, the concentration of elastase, a sensitive marker of neutrophilic activation, remained constant. The reduction of leukocytes is most probably attributable to hemodilution [36].

Thrombocytes

Chronos et al. [37] were the first to demonstrate in vitro that nonionic XCM are able to cause thrombocyte degranulation. Furthermore, an increased serotonin plasma concentration following a decrease of circulating thrombocytes in blood was observed in vivo after injection of ionic ioxaglate and nonionic iopromide [38].

Blood coagulation

Nonionic as well as ionic X-ray contrast agents engage in the blood coagulation system at various levels, they particularly inhibit fibrin polymerization and thrombocyte aggregation. However, nonionic XCM, especially at low concentrations, have markedly weaker effects than ionic XCM of high or low osmolality. The occasional observation of thrombus formation in catheters or syringes during angiographic interventions performed with nonionic XCM led to the misconception that these agents are coagulative. Nonionic contrast media are weaker anticoagulants than ionic CM but still anticoagulants. They interact less with biological processes including coagulation than ionic XCM and are, therefore, better tolerable.

Nonionic contrast media rarely and weakly react with biomacromolecules, thus the effect on prolonging blood coagulation is less marked compared with ionic XCM, as shown by blood examinations in animal models and patients [39, 40, 41]. Independently of the choice of the contrast agent the effect of catheters and syringes as well as the technical performance of the examination in terms of triggering blood coagulation through contact activation has to be observed.

**Histamine release**

The release of histamine from mastocytes in humans can trigger pseudoallergic reactions ranging from harmless skin reactions to life-threatening anaphylactoid shock.

Different nonionic XCM showed lower histamine release from rat mastocytes compared to ionic diatrizoic acid. At a contrast medium concentration of 100 mg/ml, histamine release induced by diatrizoic acid was 77 % as opposed to only 3 % for iopromide (fig. 18). In humans, the effect of XCM on histamine-packed mastocytes of the lung is lower upon rapid intra-arterial injection than upon intravenous administration.

This difference might be attributable to the fact that, after intra-arterial injection, the CM bolus passes other organs and becomes diluted before reaching the lung, whereas an i.v. bolus initially passes the lung capillaries at a high concentration.

Every contrast agent is able to increase the blood plasma's histamine level soon after injection, but only for a few minutes. This increase is not mediated by complement activation [42].

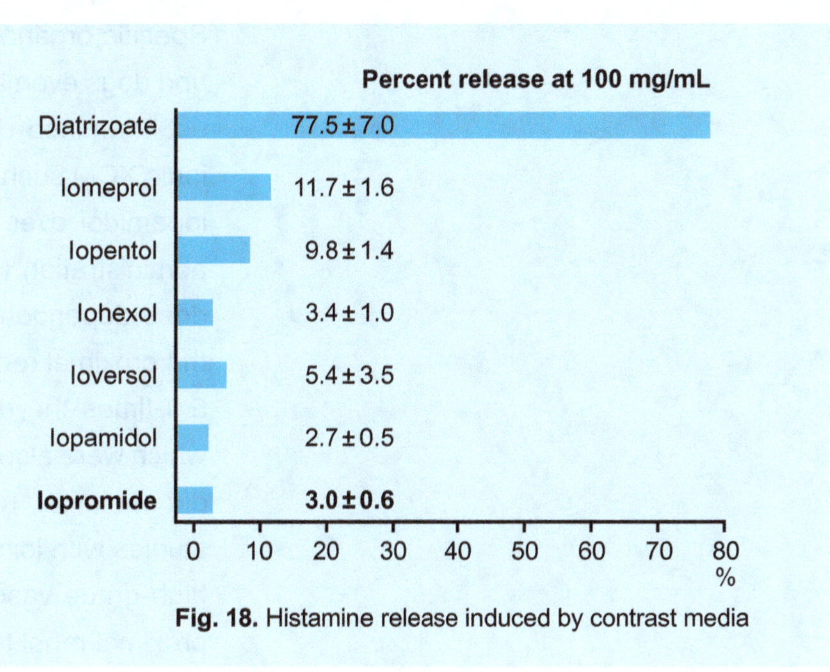


**Fig. 18.** Histamine release induced by contrast media

## Pharmacological-Toxicological Properties

For risk assessment of new iodinated X-ray contrast agents, animal experiments had to be performed before clinical trials could be initiated. The toxicological examinations correspond to those used for pharmaceuticals for single administration, i.e.

- Acute toxicity
- Systemic tolerance when applied repeatedly for approximately 4 weeks
- Genotoxicity
- Reproduction toxicity
- Local tolerance
- Examination to detect anaphylactic reactions

Iodinated nonionic XCM are usually characterized by a low acute toxicity. The LD50 for dogs, rats and mice after i.v. administration of nonionic XCM is >10 g iodine/kg. Investigations of systemic tolerance after repeated XCM administration are of great importance for risk assessment in humans. Specific organotoxic effects were not found in rats and dogs even after repeat i.v. injection of the highest examined dose ($\geq 2.4$-$\leq 4$ g iodine/kg) of nonionic XCM such as iotrolan, iohexol, iopromide and iopamidol over a period of 3-4 weeks. Repeated administration (3-5 weeks) of these XCM led to a dose-dependent vacuolization of epithelial cells of the proximal renal tubules starting at a dose of 1.4-5.0 times the diagnostic dose. Those alterations, which were also observed for ionic contrast agents, did not impair renal function. Electron-microscopic studies with ioxaglate (7.5 g iodine/kg) indicate that high-grade vascuolization of epithelial cells of the proximal renal tubule does not lead to structural alterations of cell organelles [43].

**Tolerance limits**

Contrast agents are highly concentrated aqueous solutions. A common product contains 150-400 mg I/ml, corresponding to 300-800 mg iodinated organic molecule. Based on animal experiments of acute toxicity including LD50 (mice, rats), subarachnoid administration, and vascular pain as well as extensive experiences in clinical practice, the following average and maximum doses are proposed for adults. The recommended dose of well-tolerated nonionic XCM in adults is on the order of 1-2 ml/kg body weight (BW) (maximum dose 3 ml/kg BW).

Apart from type and dose of XCM, acute toxicity is also influenced by the injection rate and pre-existing organic diseases, e.g., diabetes mellitus and renal insufficiency. This is to be taken into account when choosing the right dose.

**Effects on the cardiovascular system**

Effects on the cardiovascular system can be caused by:

- Osmolality of XCM with rapid ionic and liquid shifts
- Chemical impact on the myocardium and cardiac conduction system
- Release of vasoactive substances.

Rapid intravenous contrast agent injection has a direct impact on vascular walls, leading to vasodilatation and a drop in blood pressure with reflective tachycardia. In coronary angiocraphic examinations, high doses of the contrast agent selectively reach the myocardium, which leads to depressive dose-dependent effects on cardiac contractility.

High-osmolar CM can cause bradycardia, which lasts longer in ischemic hearts. Causes of cardiotoxic effects were investigated in experiments on dogs.

At 10-minute intervals, 0.3-0.4 ml XCM were directly injected into the aortic root of anesthetized laboratory animals until a lethal dose was reached or the experiment was aborted after 15 injections.

Solutions of ionic contrast media interfere with the ionic balance of the myocardium due to high osmolality and binding of calcium [44]. Sodium salts had the highest cardiotoxicity. In a representative experiment, it triggered ventricular fibrillation after only 1-3 injections. Nonionic XCM have lower osmolality and do not bind calcium. Therefore, they induced weaker cardiotoxic reactions such as lower influence on blood pressure in the aorta in animal experiments and are generally better tolerated in clinical coronary angiography [45].

**Influence on renal function**

Important mechanisms of nephrotoxicity are disturbances of renal perfusion and damage of glomeruli and tubular cells, which leads to proteinuria. Contrast agents cause these effects to a variable extent. Five tubular enzymes (Y-GT, ALP, LDH, AAP, N-acetyl-beta-D-glucosaminidase) showed a significant increase in activity in urine on the first day after injection of high- and low-osmolar contrast media, which indicates damage of tubular cells [46]. A significant reduction of renal blood flow was induced by 10 ml XCM solution in an isolated perfused rat kidney.

Studies on rats also showed excessive temporary decrease in renal plasma flow after injection of low-osmolar XCM with a concomitant decrease in partial oxygen pressure. No relationship with the osmolality of the contrast agent was identified [47].

Even high doses and concentrations of iodinated contrast media induce acute nephropathy in patients with normal renal function in less than 1 % of cases after i.v. injection and in 2-7 % after intra-arterial injection [48, 49]. However, XCM injection can cause further severe deterioration of renal function in patients with pre-existing renal insufficiency, especially in association with insulin-dependent diabetes, high-grade proteinuria, cardiac insufficiency and high blood pressure. The chemotoxicity of the agent as well as high osmolality and high viscosity of the solution contribute to the development of contrast medium-induced nephropathy. A (usually transient) increase in serum creatinine of more than 25 % or 44 µmol/l (0.5-1 mg/dl) or a decrease in creatinine clearance of at least 25 % during the first three days after intravascular XCM administration is considered to indicate nephrotoxicity [50].

**Allergic and pseudoallergic hypersensitivity reactions**

X-ray contrast media are chemically inert substances, of which high doses (up to > 100 g) are administered into the vascular system during a short period of time. The development of nonionic XCM has significantly improved the tolerance of these substances. Nevertheless, hypersensitivity reactions can occur [51].

Such reactions are rare and tend to be mild as the most common hypersensitivity reactions are nausea and vomiting. However, bronchospasm, life-threatening drop of blood pressure, cardiac arrest and unconsciousness may occur but are extremely rare. These reactions usually arise during the first 5-10 minutes after injection.

All hypersensitivity reactions are unrelated to the dose or osmolality of the contrast agent given. Early and late hypersensitivity reactions are distinguished (up to 1 h versus 1 h to 7 days after XCM injection).

The patient's symptoms do not allow differentiation of allergic from pseudoallergic reactions. Because nonallergic and allergic symptoms are rather similar, terms like anaphylactoid, pseudoallergic or allergy-like are used to describe these reactions.

During the occurrence of immediate hypersensitivity reactions, be it IgE-mediated allergic or nonallergic reactions, the release of histamine has a central role besides other mediators such as prostaglandins, leukotrienes and cytokines. It is known today that an IgE-mediated allergy to XCM is extremely rare [52, 53].

The molecular size and weak protein binding of nonionic contrast media almost completely prevent the formation of antibodies in vivo and even in animals under experimental conditions.

Other processes involved in the development of pseudoallergic reactions include activation of the complement system and the contact system (plasma contact system).

The release of histamine can be mediated by direct contact of contrast agents with mastocytes and basophilic granulocytes or by indirect complement activation with formation of cleavage products C3a and C5a. The active peptides C3a and C5a increase the permeability of capillaries and venules, which explains the reduction of intravascular volume during severe hypersensitivity reactions.

Administration of contrast media can lead to endothelial damage, which activates the contact system. The contact system includes the blood coagulation system, the fibrinolytic system and the prekallikrein-kallikrein system. Activation of factor XI stimulates the transformation of prekallikrein to kallikrein. Kallikrein in turn is able to cleave kinins in blood plasma, resulting in formation of the vasoactive compounds bradykinin and lysyl-bradykinin Bradykinin, for instance, inherits histamine-like characteristics.

All of these reactions are quite complex and are controlled by many factors and inhibitors. For example, the shortage of C1-esterase inhibitor seems to play a role in activation of the complement system and contact system. The enzyme C1-esterase, which activates C1, i.e., the first component of the complement system, can be inhibited by C1-esterase inhibitor.

Late hypersensitivity reactions were not encountered until the advent of nonionic dimeric contrast agents about 30 years ago [54]. These reactions are mostly mild to moderate skin reactions with and without pruritus and, less commonly, headaches, pain at the injection site, gastrointestinal conditions and flu-like symptoms.

They are most often observed between six hours and three days after i.v. administration of XCM. While such late reactions may be quite unpleasant and difficult to treat, they mostly vanish after three to seven days [55].

Different pathological mechanisms have been proposed to explain the development of late skin reactions. It is believed that most of them are T-cell-mediated reactions, an immunological type IV mechanism [56, 57].

**Endothelial damage**
Endothelial damage can occur at the injection site and other areas exposed to temporarily high contrast medium concentrations such as the blood-brain barrier in cerebral angiography or vessel segments close to stenoses in coronary or peripheral angiography. This kind of damage is primarily caused by the hyperosmolality of the contrast solution but also by its chemotoxicity. In vitro studies have shown reduced proliferation and increased apoptosis of endothelial cells after incubation of human vascular endothelial cells in intravascular XCM solutions. The effect was lowest for nonionic low-osmolar contrast media [58].

Furthermore, XCM can have temporary effects on microcirculation.

After injection of 20 ml iopromide via a subclavian artery catheter, the flow velocity of erythrocytes in finger fold capillaries decreased by 50 % for 2 minutes [59].

## Nervous system

Temporary neurotoxic effects such as convulsive conditions can occur in cerebral and spinal angiography when the blood-brain barrier is disrupted by the contrast agent or as a result of pathological conditions allowing the contrast agent to interact directly with nerve tissue. Those rare neurological effects are related to the chemical structure of the contrast agent rather than physicochemical characteristics such as osmolality or viscosity of the contrast medium solution.

A considerable proportion of neurological problems is attributable to the technical execution of the catheter examination and not so much to the use of ionic or nonionic XCM [60, 61].

Neurotoxicity in animals was investigated by assessing damage to the blood-brain barrier after contrast medium administration for cerebral angiography. After direct injection of the contrast agent into a cerebral ventricle alterations in EEG, behavior and other neural activities are observed.

In studies on rabbits, slight blood-brain barrier damage was demonstrated for the nonionic, monomeric agents iohexol and ioversol and for the nonionic, dimeric agents iodixanol and iotrolan using technetium-99m-pertechnetate as a tracer. A hyperosmolar mannitol solution of 714 mosm/kg showed less damage, indicating the additional role of chemotoxicity [62].

EEG alterations observed in sedated rabbits after intracerebral injection of iopromide and iohexol differed only lightly between the two agents and did not show any statistically significant difference compared with the effects of an isosmotic mannitol solution [63].

## Pharmacokinetics

Two groups of XCM are distinguished on the basis of their pharmacokinetic behavior in the human body: contrast agents that are excreted by the kidneys (CM for computed tomography (CT), angiography and urography) and distribute in the intravascular and extracellular fluid space and hepatocellular or tissue-specific contrast agents (CM for choleangiography).

The water-soluble, iodinated contrast agents used for CT and angiography are not able to pass cell membranes and are mainly eliminated renally. They are not enterally resorbed. After intravascular injection, contrast agents distribute only passively with the blood stream. Their binding to plasma proteins is quite minor (<5%). They enter the interstitial space of most tissues through pores in the capillary wall. Distribution in the intravascular space lasts about 2-3 minutes, whereas the diffusion in the interstitium takes about 10-30 minutes [64]. Contrast agents are eliminated unchanged from the blood through glomerular filtration with an elimination half-life of about 1.5-2 hours.

A much longer elimination half-life of up to 10 hours may be observed in patients with renal insufficiency, which reduces renal clearance to 20 ml/min and less. Nevertheless, complete elimination was shown for the nonionic iopamidol [65].

Hemodialysis is an effective and safe means to accelerate contrast medium excretion from the body in patients with severe renal insufficiency.

Contrast agents including the cholegraphic media are not able to pass an intact blood-brain barrier. Passage of the placenta and transition into breast milk is markedly restricted.

A very small proportion of iodine is released from water-soluble, iodinated contrast agents in the human body, even though iodine is strongly bound to the benzene ring. The amount of iodide released from contrast media may reach 3-10 mg per use. There is virtually no risk of interference with thyroid function in healthy patients; however, serious problems may occur in patients with hyperthyroidism. Nevertheless, in all patients, the radioactive iodine uptake test may be altered for weeks after administration of XCM.

The common i.v. choleangiographic agents are composed of two chemically covalently connected tri-iodinated benzoic acid derivates ("dimers"). The molecules are therefore large enough for biliary elimination. The minimum molecular weight for biliary elimination is about 400 Dalton (calculated without the heavy, but small iodine atoms). Intravenous cholegraphics surpass this size without forming conjugates with glucuronic acid whereas the increase in molecular weight through glucuronidation is required for so many other biliarily eliminated substances in the human body and also for the smaller oral cholecystographic agents.

During adequately slow i.v. infusion (10-20 min), iotroxic acid (Biliscopin) is bound to plasma proteins to 80-90 % and is thereby protected from glomerular filtration. A dose of 5 g iodine is sufficient for ensuring biliary clearance for a minimum of one hour at a maximum transport rate of 0.4 mg/kg BW/min in patients with intact liver function. In these patients, 90 % of the contrast agent dose is excreted via feces and only 10 % through the kidneys. XCM reaching the intestine with the bile is not resorbed.

# USES OF X-RAY CONTRAST MEDIA

The mechanisms of action of X-ray CM range from purely mechanical filling of certain cavities to opacification in a functional manner.

Functional opacification exploits the physiologic function of organs, such as the kidneys and liver, namely the elimination of metabolic endproducts or exogenous substances, to visualize the organ or its drainage pathways.

The most common uses of XCM are imaging of arteries and veins and enhancement of contrasts between tissues based on differences in blood volume, perfusion, capillary permeability, and size of the interstitial space (table 12 a-c).

## Modes of opacification

The identification of morphological structures is the main objective of direct luminal filling via a natural or iatrogenically (e.g., by puncture) created access; this permits the differentiation of superficial or mural changes. In addition, this mode of opacification can provide functional information, e.g., assessment of changes in tone or peristalsis in hollow passages (GI tract, ureters with retrograde filling, etc.) (fig. 19).

| Modes of opacification | Example | CM characteristics |
|---|---|---|
| **Luminal filling** | | No absorption; mild or no toxicity |
| G.I. tract | Retrograde pyelography | |
| **Organ function** | Blood vessel | Organ-specific accumulation and elimination |
| Cholegraphy | i.v. urography | |
| **Parenchymal staining (enhancement)** | | CM distribution dependent on circulation |
| Liver CT | Kidney | |
| **Angiography** | | Special physico-chemical properties (osmolality, viscosity) |
| CT angiography | | |

**Fig. 19.** Modes of opacification

In cavography, the concentration of the CM administered is decisive for the degree of contrast in the radiograph. In urography and cholegraphy, on the other hand, contrast density is essentially dependent on the functional capacity of the organs being examined. Consequently, assessment of both function and morphology is possible after CM administration.

Thus, the radiological evaluation of the kidneys and turinary tract or of the hepatobiliary system reveals both morphologic and functional changes of the respective organs.

The additional functional information can provide important clues for the differential diagnosis. For example, delayed elimination of renal CM can be interpreted to indicate impaired glomerular filtration due to an acute or chronic disease.

Another mode of action of XCM has gained importance in computed tomography: The transit and selective accumulation of CM in different organs or tissues (enhancement) improve the differentiation of morphological structures, particularly between normal and pathological tissue. This allows or at least facilitates the demonstration of pathological processes and occasionally of their etiology as well.

Fast multislice spiral CT and multi-detector CT, combined with fast image postprocessing, permits 3-dimensional imaging of the coronary arteries and other vessels after rapid i.v. injection of non-ionic contrast agents. This modality can replace invasive catheter-based angiography performed for diagnostic purposes alone.

Dynamic CT during the first pass of CM provides functional information based on pharmacokinetic behavior including contrast medium arrival, wash-out, and distribution.

In angiography, selective opacification can be achieved by direct CM injection into the vessel of interest, followed by evaluation of CM distribution and filling patterns including gaps in opacification of the target anatomy.

This evaluation yields detailed diagnostic information regarding normal and abnormal morphology and function.

| Mode of opacification | Method | Contrast agent | Dose (ml) | Iodine concentration |
|---|---|---|---|---|
| Filling of the lumen | 1. Gastrointestinal tract Orally, projection imaging | $BaSO_4$ +$CO_2$ | 150 (-400) variable | - - |
| | | Nephrotrophic CM | 50-100 | 370 300 300/370 300/350 300/350 |
| | | Nephrotrophic CM | 500-1000 | 10-20 |
| | | Nephrotrophic CM | 800-2000 | 5-14 |
| | 2. Arthrography | Nephrotrophic CM + Air | 2-10 15-35 | 300 |
| | 3. Hysterosalpingography | Nephrotrophic CM | 5-10 | 300 |
| | 4. Fistulography | Nephrotrophic CM | variable | 300 |
| | 5. Sialography | Nephrotrophic CM | 1-3 | 300 |
| | 6. PTC*, ERCP** | Nephrotrophic CM | 20-40 (10-40) | 300 |
| | 7. Retrograde Pyelography, Cystography | Nephrotrophic CM | 10-15 (100-300) 2-300 2-20 10-20 | 150 240/300/370 300 |
| | 8. Myelography | Nephrotrophic CM | 15 5-15 4-12 10-15 | 240-300 200/300 240 240 |

**Table. 12a.** Overview of contrast media uses

| Mode of opacification | Method | Contrast agent | Dose (ml) |
|---|---|---|---|
| **Organ function** | 1. i.v. Urography | Nephrotrophic CM | 50-100 |
| | 2. Inf. Urography | Nephrotrophic CM | (250) |
| | 3. i.v. Cholegraphy | Liver passing CM | 20-30 |
| **Parenchymal enhancement** | 1. Bolusinjection | Nephrotrophic CM | 1 ml/Kg BW p.r.n. more |
| | 2. Infusion | | 50-125 |

**Table. 12b.** Overview of contrast media uses; * PTC: percutaneous transhepatic cholangiography, ** ERCP: endoscopic retrograde cholangiopancreatography

| Commercial preparations/ Trademark/ Type of contrast agent | Comments |
| --- | --- |
| HD preparations<br>Micropaque<br>$CO_2$ | Hypotonia due to butylscopolamine (20 mg i.v. or i.m.)<br>Faster gastrointestinal passage due to Paspertin |
| Gastrografin<br>Isovist<br>Ultravist<br>Omnipaque<br>Imagopaque | No barium in patients with (suspected) perforation/ suture insufficiency |
| Gastrografin 30-40 ml/L<br><br>Accupaque | For CT: fractionated administration 30 min – 6 h before examination if necessary |
| Isovist,<br>Ultravist,<br>Solutrast,<br>Omnipaque,<br>Imagopaque,<br>Imeron etc. | |
| Ultravist etc. | |
| Omnipaque,<br>Solutrast,<br>Imeron | |
| Isovist etc. | |
| Telebrix<br>Urografin 30 %<br>Ultravist<br>Imeron | |
| Isovist<br>Iopamiron<br>Accupaque<br>Optitray | Iodine concentration of 200-300 mg/ml |

| Iodine concentration | Commercial preparations/ Trademark/ Type of contrast agent | Comments |
| --- | --- | --- |
| 300 | Ultravist, | Dehydrogenation is dispensable with nonionic CM |
| 150-300 | Omnipaque<br>Solutrast etc. | |
| 180 | | Injector for constant flow |
| 300-370 | Omnipaque<br>Solutrast | Administration directly before the examination. Scan series begins approximately 20 sec after start of injection |
| 150-370 | Ultravist etc. | |

| Mode of imaging | Method | Contrast agent | Dose (ml) |
|---|---|---|---|
| **Conventional Vasography** | 1. Cardioangiography | Nephrotrophic CM | 40-60 |
| | 2. Coronary angiography | Nephrotrophic CM | 5-8 |
| | 3. Angiography | Nephrotrophic CM | 50 |
| | 4. Selective abdominal angiography | Nephrotrophic CM | 5-50 |
| | 5. Angiography of the Extremities | Nephrotrophic CM nonionic | 10-70 |
| | 6. Cerebral angiography | Nephrotrophic CM nonionic | 5-10 |
| | 7. Phlebography | Nephrotrophic CM | 40 |
| | 8. IA DSA | Nephrotrophic CM | As conventional angiography |
| | 9. Direct lymphography | Oily | 5-10 per extrememity |

**Table. 12c.** Overview of contrast uses

Digital subtraction angiography (DSA) allows selective evaluation of arteries and veins without interfering background (e.g., bone) and with a very much lower CM concentration in the vascular regions of interest.

DSA is based on the subtraction of an image obtained immediately before CM injection from a series of images obtained with maximum CM filling of the target vessels.

In DSA, electronic amplification of only slight differences between the precontrast and the contrast-enhanced images results in images highlighting vessel contrast.

| Iodine concentration | Commercial preparations/ Trademark/ Type of contrast agent | Comments |
| --- | --- | --- |
| 370 | Omnipaque | |
| 370 | Solutrast<br>Ultravist etc. | |
| 300-370 | | |
| 300 | Omnipaque<br>Solutrast<br>Ultravist etc. | Dose, CM concentration and injection rate have to be the higher the better the spatial resolution, the faster the blood flow, and the larger the distance between the catheter tip and the vascular target territory is. |
| 300 | | |
| 300 | | |
| 150-300 | Omnipaque<br>Solutrast<br>Ultravist etc. | |
| 75-300 | As conventional angiography | Less selective injection or smaller volume or lower iodine concentration is possible due to higher sensitivity of DSA |
| 480 | Lipiodol | Administration into lymphatic vessels |

In addition, electronic data processing speeds up postprocessing of the DSA images, so that the results are immediately available.

DSA allows evaluation of larger arteries even after i.v. bolus injection of CM. In i.v. DSA and fast CT, high doses and rapid injection make particularly great demands on the tolerance of the CM. For more details see table 12 a,b and c.

# INTERACTIONS

## Influence on laboratory tests

The influence of different ionic and nonionic CM on clinicochemical parameters determined in serum and urine was examined systematically in the laboratory.

For this purpose, reference sera (normal and pathological values) were mixed with up to 20 vol% CM solution and urine with up to 50% CM solution. Higher concentrations are unlikely to occur in humans even a very short time after a CM injection.

In this investigation, Ultravist, Urografin (diatrizoate) and iohexol did not affect serum levels of GOT GPT, Y-GT, AP, LDH, HBDH, CK, CKMB, ChE, GDH, amylase (with maltotetraose, Biomed) and lipase (Automatic Clinical Analyzer, Du Pont). Meglumine sodium ioxaglate caused suppression of GPT.

Similarly, the urinary enzymes Y-GT, LDH, AAP, ß-NAG and amylase were not or only slightly influenced by the above CM. The specific gravity of urine was found to increase after administration of iodinated renal CM.

Protein determination by the biuret assay was not affected by Ultravist, while marked effects were observed for some other CM investigated. No effects on protein levels in urine were observed using the Ponceau S method.


U. Speck, *X-Ray Contrast Media*, https://doi.org/10.1007/978-3-662-56465-3_9

Levels of the substrates BUN, creatinine, uric acid, bilirubin (direct and indirect), glucose, cholesterol and triglycerides were not appreciably affected by Ultravist. In contrast, other CM led to, at times marked, changes in individual parameters. Electrolytes (particularly iron and copper) were affected by all CM tested and very much so by some. Whenever an effect cannot be ruled out with certainty, samples for serum or urinary analysis should be obtained either before CM administration or at the earliest 24 hours afterwards. In patients with severe renal failure and hence delayed CM elimination, it may be necessary to wait even longer.

All tests concerning the thyroid gland can be disturbed for much longer than 24 hours by the iodide administered with the CM. The ability of the thyroid tissue to take up radioisotopes for the diagnosis of thyroid disease is reduced by iodinated CM for 2-6 weeks. Urographic CM affect laboratory test results least, while orally administered cholegraphic agents and iodinated oily CM have a longer-lasting effect.

To date, only a few interactions of CM for urography, angiography and CT with medications have been described in association with clinical use. Such interactions are extremely improble since these CM bind hardly at all to plasma proteins, cause no inhibition of enzymes, are not themselves subject to metabolism, and are not absorbed enterally. In cancer patients treated with interleukin-2, more side-effects have been observed after administration of ionic and nonionic contrast media. These side-effects include fever, nausea, vomiting, skin reactions, and diarrhea [66]. On the other hand, butylscopolamine appears to have no influence on contrast medium tolerance [67].

Due to the risk of lactate acidosis it was originally recommended that treatment with biguanides (Glucophage, Metformin) should be withdrawn two days before administration of intravascular X-ray contrast media to avoid accumulation of the exclusively renally excreted Metformin should the contrast medium induce renal failure [68]. This risk would also be eliminated if biguanide therapy were withdrawn from after contrast medium administration until an effect on kidney function can be ruled out [69].

A variety of pharmaceutical substances were tested for their influence on acute tolerance of CM in animal experiments. Even here, interactions possibly of clinical relevance were rarely observed [70, 71]. In cardioangiography, there is a theoretical concern that the cardiodepressive effect of ionic CM caused by calcium binding will be intensified by calcium blockers (verapamil) [72].

One case of thrombotic occlusion of the leg arteries which could not be alleviated with continuous urokinase infusion has been reported in the literature [73]. Patients with cardiac insufficiency and renal dysfunction undergoing angiography should not be given furosemide (diuretic) − even with large quantities of liquid. Patients who received 110 mg furosemide along with 3 liters of fluid exhibited a creatinine rise from $145 \pm 13$ to $182 \pm 16\,\mu mol/l$, whereas controls without furosemide showed no rise [74].

There is also evidence that neuroleptic agents (chlorpromazine) potentiate the normally only slight epileptogenic effect even of nonionic CM in myelography [75].

Cholegraphic agents bind to plasma proteins and are eliminated with the bile via an active transport mechanism which is limited in its capacity. They are able to displace drugs and endogenous substances that have the same properties. In this way, the concentrations of free drug in plasma can be increased by the simultaneous administration of biliary CM and their excretion delayed to some extent. The absorption of oral cholegraphic agents relies on their passage from the stomach into the bowel. Drugs which affect the gastric passage of these agents, therefore, alter the rate of their absorption.

The same effect is likely to occur in the presence of substances or foodstuffs which have an influence on the absorption of pharmaceutical substances from the bowel (e.g., carbon, gel-forming substances, fats, and coffee).

In the course of some diagnostic or interventional radiological procedures, X-ray contrast media are treated in a special manner, mixed with therapeutic agents, or come into contact with high local concentrations of equally undiluted drugs in the body. This may result in precipitation of the contrast medium, the therapeutic agent, or both, inactivation of the drugs, or occurrence of other undesirable and sometimes hardly predictable effects (table 13).

| Active agent | Diatrizoic Acid | Ioxaglate | Iopromide |
|---|---|---|---|
| Heating of the CM up to 100° C e.g. for the purpose of embolization | possible | possible | possible |
| Compound with ethanol | ? | ? | possible |
| | | | |
| Mixing before injection | | | |
| Papaverine | + | + | - |
| Phentolamine mesylate | + | + | - |
| Tolazolin | - | - | - |
| Diphenhydramine | + | + | - |
| Prostaglandin E1 | - | - | - |
| Pheniramin | - | - | - |
| Cimetidine | + | + | - |
| Na-heparin | - | - | - |
| Protamine | + | + | - |
| Vasopressin | - | - | - |
| Epinephrine | - | - | - |
| Hydrocortisone Na-succinate | - | - | - |
| Methylprednisolone Na-succinate[a] | - | - | - |
| Lidocaine | - | - | - |
| Diazepam | + | - | - |
| Nitroglycerin | - | - | - |
| Benzylpenicillin | - | - | - |
| Ampicillin | - | - | - |
| Erythromycin[a] | - | - | - |
| Gentamicin | - | + | - |
| Chloramphenicol | - | - | - |
| Urokinase | - | - | - |

+=Solution stays clear , -=Solution precipitates
*=50% loss off efficiacy when adding iopromide corresponding 170mg Iodine/ml

**Table. 13.** Data on interactions found in literature [76, 77]

## Effects on blood coagulation

Nonionic contrast media come closer to the ideal of completely pharmacologically inert substances than ionic contrast media. Ionic contrast media inhibit enzymes involved with blood coagulation as well as other processes more strongly than nonionic X-ray contrast media.

Ionic X-ray contrast media are
- more anticoagulative [78]

Nonionic X-ray contrast media are
- less anticoagulative [78]

| Sample | Coagulation time in sec. |
|---|---|
| Plasma without additives | 11  (10.5–10.9) |
| Plasma + physiol. NaCl | 12  (11.9–12.0) |
| + Angiografin | 68  (68.0–69.5) |
| + Ultravist-300 | 17  (16.4–16.8) |

**Table 14.** Thromboplastin time of human plasma without and with the addition of 25 volume percent test solution; n = 4, mean and 95 % confidence limits

The anticoagulative effect of contrast is viewed by some radiologists as additional protection against thrombus formation during imperfect performance of catheter angiography.

Laboratory examinations have shown significant differences in the anticoagulative effect of ionic (e.g., Angiografin) and nonionic contrast media (Ultravist) (table 14). The addition of small quantities of heparin to nonionic X-ray contrast media ensures effective inhibition of blood coagulation, similar to that characteristic of ionic contrast media (fig. 20). It was shown that 5 IU heparin/ml Ultravist is sufficient to completely suppress the formation of thrombi under standard experimental conditions. Even with a volume of 300 ml heparinized contrast medium, no systemic anticoagulative effects should be expected. The good tolerance of the nonionic contrast medium remains unchanged.

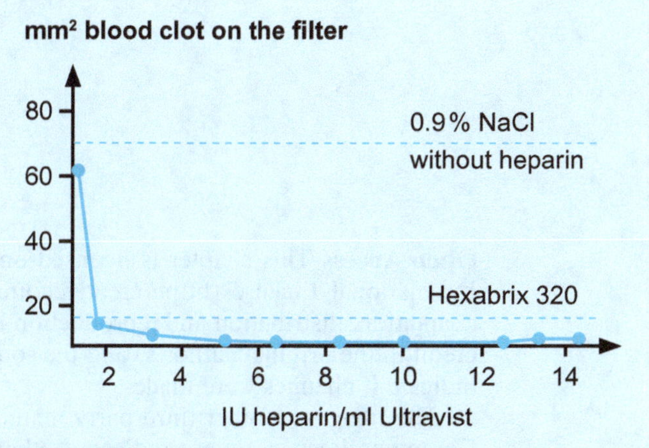


**Fig. 20.** Size of blood clots after 90 min. Incubation of 2 ml human blood in 10 ml plastic syringes with 5 ml test solution; not mixed, maximum contact surface

# RISKS OF CONTRAST MEDIA USE

The aim of using CM is to visualize certain structures in the organism or improve their visualization and to obtain information on organ functions. A CM must have low toxicity and be safe to use since it is often injected at a high dose and for certain purposes very quickly.

## Barium sulfate

Barium sulfate is insoluble in water and usually safe when administered orally or rectally for imaging the intestine. While barium ions are toxic, the small amounts present in the suspension of the insoluble barium sulfate and available for intestinal absorption can normally be ignored. Serious complications after barium examinations of the upper and lower GI tracts are few [79]. There are, however, some patients at risk in whom barium sulfate should not be used because of possible aspiration or suspected perforation. Once barium sulfate enters the lungs or leaks from the stomach or intestine, excretion is impossible or very slow and persistent inflammation causes severe problems. Some of the most serious adverse effects after administration of barium preparations are:

- Retention of barium in the colon for some weeks or longer in elderly patients or patients with partial colonic obstruction
- Formation of barium fecoliths, sometimes seen in diverticula of the colon
- Leakage of barium into the peritoneal cavity
- Aspiration of barium into the bronchial tree
- Hypersensitivity reactions to barium preparations, caused by the additives of the barium preparations [80].



U. Speck, *X-Ray Contrast Media*, https://doi.org/10.1007/978-3-662-56465-3_10

| Kind of examination | No. of patients | Incidence of side effects (%) | No. of deaths |
| --- | --- | --- | --- |
| Urography | 214,033 | 10,257 (4.80) | 11 |
| Cholagiography | 33,778 | 2,676 (8.00) | 2 |
| Cerebral angiography | 12,771 | 263 (2.06) | 1 |
| Angiocardiography | 7,911 | 179 (2.26) | 2 |
| Aortography | 24,885 | 665 (2.67) | 1 |
| Other angiographies | 2,815 | 101 (3.58) | 0 |
| Venography | 5,890 | 160 (2.72) | 1 |
| **Total** | **302,083** | **14,301 (4.73)** | **18 (0.006%)** |

**Table. 15.** Incidence of side effects in various CM examinations [81] using ionic CM

## Ionic contrast media

Extensive statistics are available on the side effects of ionic CM. The incidence of reactions depends on a large number of factors, such as the patient's general condition, the kind of examination (table 15), the type of CM, its dose, and also the conditions under which the examination is being conducted. Special attention has been devoted to the frequency of severe and fatal CM incidents. While available data (table 16) diverge greatly, taken together, they suggest that, with the ionic preparations, fatal CM incidents are very rare events, given the frequency of use of these substances.

| | | | |
| --- | --- | --- | --- |
| 1 : | 116,000 | Pendergrass, USA | 1960 |
| 1 : | 85,000 | Toniolo, Italy | 1966 |
| 1 : | 61,000 | Wolfromm, France | 1966 |
| 1 : | 40,000 | Ansell, U.K. | 1970 |
| 1 : | 54,000 | Fischer, USA | 1972 |
| 1 : | 30,000 | Witten, USA | 1973 |
| 1 : | 10,000 | Shehadi, USA | 1975 |
| 1 : | 20,000 | Shehadi, USA | 1980 |
| 1 : | 75,000 | Hartmann, USA | 1982 |

**Table. 16.** Risk of death with i.v. urography

## Nonionic contrast media

Nonionic contrast media are much better tolerated than ionic contrast media in many ways (table 17). A number of trials investigated the frequency of general reactions after intravenous administration of nonionic X-ray contrast media (table 18), some of them in comparison to conventional ionic X-ray contrast media. The available data allow general statements regarding the frequency of severe reactions but it is not possible to provide sound information on the frequency of deaths related to the use of nonionic contrast media. However, it is very likely that nonionic X-ray contrast media are less frequently related to fatalities or life-threatening conditions (unconsciousness of the patient, conditions requiring an anesthetist etc.) than ionic contrast media (table 18).

On the other hand, it must be borne in mind that all of the known types of side-effects associated with ionic contrast media can also occur during the administration of nonionic contrast media. Only the frequency has actually changed. One must, therefore, always be prepared to treat contrast medium reactions.

|  | Conventional ionic X-ray-CM | Low osmolar ionic X-ray-CM | Nonionic X-Ray-CM |
|---|---|---|---|
| General reactions (nausea, vomiting, allergoid side-effects, some cardiovascular reactions) | ▼ | ▼ | ▲ |
| Neural tolerance | ▼ | ▼ | ▲ |
| Osmolality-dependent effects (pain, vasodilation, bradycardia, diuresis etc.) | ▼ | ▲ | ▲ |
| Calcium binding (cardiodepression) | ▼ | ▼ | ▲ |
| General renal tolerance, i.v. | ● | ● | ● |
| Renal arteriography | ▼ | ● | ▲ |

▼ poorly tolerated　　▲ much better tolerated　　● no significant difference or difference not proven

**Table. 17.** Differences in tolerance between the individual types of X-ray contrast media for urography, angiography and CT

| Trial | Nonionic CM side-effects | | Ionic CM side-effects | |
|---|---|---|---|---|
|  | total | severe/very severe | total | severe/very severe |
| Schrott [82] 50,660 cases | 2.1% | 0.01% |  |  |
| Palmer [83] 30,228 nonionic cases 79,278 ionic cases | 1.2% | 0.02% | 3.8% | 0.09% |
| Katayama [6] 168,363 nonionic cases 169,284 ionic cases | 3.1% | 0.04% | 12.7% | 0.22% |
| Cochran [84] 73,039 nonionic cases 12,916 inonic cases | 0.3% | 0.02% | 1.3% | 0.05% |

**Table. 18.** Frequency of side-effects related to i.v. injection of nonionic and ionic X-ray contrast media (severe/very severe reaction requires that the patient be immediately hospitalized)

## Delayed reactions

Following the introduction of nonionic contrast media, reactions have been reported which are first noticed hours or even days after administration.

A comparative study of iohexol and iopamidol was performed in 2,382 patients undergoing CT examinations.

Reactions delayed by up to 2 days were twice as common as reactions occurring in the first 30 minutes. Headache and rash were the most frequent delayed reactions. Although all delayed reactions were mild in intensity, the attending physician should inform the patient about the possibility of delayed reactions [85].

A greater frequency of allergy-like delayed reactions was observed for intravascular administration of nonionic dimeric X-ray contrast media. These also included rare severe events lasting for several days and requiring therapy. The causes, risk factors, mechanisms of action, and the actual frequency especially of severe delayed hypersensitivity reactions remain unknown despite concerted efforts to elucidate them [86].

## Causes of contrast media reactions

Contrast medium side-effects generally cannot be explained by a single mechanism [87]. The type of contrast agent and its particular pharmacological properties, the examination technique employed, such as the magnitude of the dose and the mode of administration, and finally, the patient's attitude, such as fear, are all regarded as important contributing factors. CM side effects can be classified in several ways, but the most appropriate is by their cause.

Classification by cause:
- General or largely dose-independent CM reactions (anaphylaxis).
- Chemotoxic, local and cardiovascular effects, dose-dependent side-effects (concentration. volume).

## General reactions (anaphylactoid reactions)

General or largely dose-independent CM reactions range from mild reactions, such as urticaria, to moderately severe reactions, such as bronchospasm, and severe reactions, such as collapse or even cardiac arrest, to fatal outcome. Severe and fatal reactions are rare. The mortality reported for conventional ionic CM is one out of 10,000 to 100,000 patients.

These reactions may occur in any patient without any warning. Because of this, the attending physician must be prepared for all emergency measures, ranging from medications to artificial respiration.

General CM reactions have little or nothing to do with the osmolality of the CM. They can occur after administration of very small amounts of diluted and even isotonic CM.

They are observed most frequently after i.v. administration, but also in arteriography and other examination procedures.

General CM reactions have been attributed to the following underlying mechanisms:
- Effects on plasma protein, the complement system, blood coagulation, and/or vascular endothelium
- Effects mediated by the central nervous system
- Cross-reaction of the CM with antibodies which were not, however, originally formed against the CM.

## Prophylaxis of general reactions

It is now generally accepted that nonionic CM cause such reactions considerably less frequently than ionic CM and, in particular, less frequently than the low-osmolar, ionic compound meglumine sodium ioxaglate [88, 89].

Even patients who have exhibited repeat and predictable reactions to the injection of ionic CM often tolerate nonionic CM without symptoms [90]. Prophylactic effects regarding general CM reactions to both conventional ionic and nonionic preparations have been demonstrated for certain therapeutic regimes, e.g., oral administration of 32 mg methylprednisolone (*2 tablets methylprednisolone, 16 mg) 6-12 and 2 hours before the examination or the combined administration of H1 (**H1 blocker: dimethindene maleate; intravenous injection of 0.2 mg/kg BW) and H2 blockers (***H2 blocker: cimetidine; intravenous injection of 5 mg/kg BW) [91, 92, 93]. Prophylaxis aims at reducing the frequency of anaphylactoid reactions; however, it is not possible to fully eliminate such reactions by the suggested measures. It can also not be expected that the frequency or severity of any reactions other than anaphylactoid side effects (e.g., neural, renal, most cardiovascular reactions or pain) will be reduced by prophylactic treatment of patients with corticoids or histamine receptor blockers before CM administration.

In patients at risk (patients with allergic and cardiopulmonary conditions), prophylaxis with H1 and H2 blockers reduces the frequency of side-effects, even when nonionic X-ray contrast media are administered, while patients without risk factors have no benefits from H1 and H2 blockers [94]. What is certain is that calm and assured management of patients and distraction of their attention during the examination can help to avoid side effects.

## Dose-dependent side effects

Distinctly dose-dependent side effects include sensations of pain and heat, some circulatory disturbances, and renal impairment. These adverse effects are attributable to the osmolality and pharmacological properties of the agent, and it is not always possible to differentiate between these two components. All nonionic CM have markedly lower osmolality than conventional ionic contrast agents, which is one reason why they have replaced ionic contrast media to a significant degree.

The advantages of nonionic CM are especially obvious in:
• Pain-intensive applications, since osmolality is the main factor determining the painfulness of a contrast medium.
• Angiographic examinations with high total dosages from a number of single injections, e.g., cardioangiography, femoral arteriography, conventional angiography of several vascular regions, i.v. DSA, and angioplasty.

The kidney, which eliminates the CM for several hours after the examination, is regarded as the critical organ in such examinations. Effects of the nonionic CM Ultravist on renal function were examined in various clinical trials. Renal function was not recognizably impaired in any of the patients examined. The cardiovascular effects of conventional ionic CM are largely attributable to their high osmolality:
• Vasodilatation, reduction of peripheral resistance, and a decrease of blood pressure.
• Hypervolemia.
• Bradycardia in cardioangiography.

Nonionic CM have less of an influence on the heart and circulation.

When iodinated CM are administered, a healthy thyroid gland can adjust to an iodide surplus in a host of ways without increasing hormone production.

In a diseased thyroid, these selfregulating mechanisms can fail to function. In this way, a diagnostic or therapeutic iodine administration can result in severe metabolic dysfunctions such as decompensated hyperthyroidism and thyrotoxic crisis. A special risk exists for goiter patients (struma) and patients with hyperthyroidism in general. For this reason, iodinated CM should not be administered before hyperthyroidism has been ruled out. According to our present state of knowledge, the risk that hyperthyroidism will develop is not diminished by nonionic CM such as Ultravist.

The risk of hyperthyroidism is exclusively determined by the iodine and/or iodide contents of the CM. Osmolality and possible chemically toxic properties do not play any role. The renal, water-soluble, ionic and nonionic X-ray CM – as a result of the way they are produced – contain only traces of iodide, and very little of the stable chemically bonded iodine is released in the organism. Nevertheless, even these small amounts can result in further functional deterioration of a severely damaged thyroid gland (e.g., with manifest hyperthyroidism).

A peculiarity of iodine-induced hyperthyroidism is that deterioration customarily does not occur immediately but weeks or months after iodine administration.

If diagnostic measures make it essential to use iodinated CM in a patient with hyperthyroidism, combined perchlorate and carbimazole (or thiamizole)
should be given for prophylaxis. Administration of
perchlorate (3x300mg daily, from 1-2 days before
until 1 week after CM administration) inhibits the absorption of iodide by the thyroid gland; administration of methimazole simultaneously blocks hormone
synthesis (2x20mg thiamizole daily, from 1-2 days
before until 2-3 weeks after CM administration).

The longer retention times of biliary CM require a
further 3 weeks of treatment with half the dose of
thiamizole (carbimazole) [95].

## Renal damage

Ionic and nonionic contrast media used in urography, angiography and computed tomography (CT)
are eliminated mainly via the kidneys. Isolated cases of reduced kidney function including acute renal
failure following intravenous and intra-arterial administration have been described in the literature.

However, the risks related to intravenous administration in patients without obvious risk factors has
been, to some extent, exaggerated in the past.
Systematic comparative studies [96, 97] showed
that spontaneous changes in kidney function in patients who had received no contrast media were
not significantly less common than in patients receiving contrast media, e.g., for CT.

### Renal insufficiency

When ionic CM is administered intravenously for
urography in patients with healthy kidneys, deterioration in renal function is hardly ever observed; it
seems to be, however, somewhat more frequent in
those with renal insufficiency.

Deterioration is defined as an increase of 1 mg/dl in serum creatinine. Nonionic CM are well tolerated by the kidneys of patients with reduced renal function – e.g., after administering iopromide intravenously – and several trials identified no clinically relevant changes in the parameters describing renal tolerance: serum creatinine, creatinine clearance, and urinary protein. Well-designed clinical studies demonstrated that natural fluctuations of serum creatinine occur to the same extent in patients who received no CM [98, 99, 100].

In arteriography, part of the CM can flow directly into the kidneys in almost undiluted form. Under these conditions, impairment of renal function is more likely, even though nonionic CM have been better tolerated, especially in renal arteriography, than ionic CM [101].

**Plasmocytoma**

Disturbed renal function is found in a high percentage of patients with multiple myeloma. Isolated cases of acute renal failure in myeloma patients following urography have been reported in the literature. Almost all of these patients presented additional risk factors prior to CM administration, such as severe dehydration and/or sepsis. In addition, almost all of these urographic examinations were performed decades ago with diiodinated CM. In more recent retrospective studies of patients with confirmed multiple myeloma who underwent intravenous urography, no temporal connection could be established between deterioration of renal function and CM administration. In the opinion of experts, given adequate hydration and the use of modern CM, plasmocytoma is no a priori contraindication for CM administration.

Rather, more recent studies suggest that the principal risk factors for acute renal damage in patients with multiple myeloma are hypercalcemia, dehydration, infections, and Bence Jones proteinuria [102]. Patients with serum creatinine levels above 2 mg % should not undergo urography.

## Diabetes mellitus

Proteinuria and elevated serum creatinine in patients with insulin-dependent diabetes mellitus indicate advanced diabetic glomerular sclerosis. These patients are more likely to show deterioration in renal function after CM administration. As a rule, only severe proteinuria (300 mg/24 h) will significantly increase the risk of acute renal failure in a diabetes mellitus patient. In this condition, high concentrations of dissolved materials contained in urine tend to precipitate in the presence of CM and may cause tubular blockage.

## Prophylaxis

Patients with risk factors for reduced renal tolerance should not receive high intravascular doses of contrast media. These risk factors include
• limited renal function in conjunction with
• a long history of insulin-dependent diabetes
  mellitus,
• cardiac insufficiency,
• and advanced age.

Several alternative imaging modalities including ultrasound, magnetic resonance imaging, and arterial digital subtraction angiography are available to avoid or diminish the use of X-ray contrast media in these patients.

The following prophylactic measures are recommended to reduce the risk of renal damage [103]:

- ensure adequate hydration by sufficient water intake
- avoid multiple examinations with X-ray contrast media during a short period of only a few days
- discontinue medications which might impair renal function

A recommendation for medical prophylaxis adequately confirmed by clinical studies cannot at present be made. A possible prophylactic effect is known primarily for theophylline. However, the optimal dose for prevention of CIN has not been established [104].

## Pregnant patients

The use of CM during pregnancy has not yet been proven to be harmless although toxicological studies in animals and clinical experience do not indicate any particular risk. Since exposure to radiation should be avoided during this period, the potential risks of any X-ray examination must be given careful consideration.

## Breast-feeding mothers

Only very small proportions of renal CM and i.v. cholegraphic agents enter breast milk. They are barely reabsorbed in breast-feeding so that one can assume that there is no danger to the infant. Even with oral cholecystographic agents, exposure of the infant is minimal.

## Pheochromocytoma

Patients with pheochromocytoma often undergo X-ray examinations prior to surgery to determine the site, size, and number of tumors. Such examinations are not totally without risk to patients. In angiography, especially with selective CM injection into tumor vessels, a spontaneous release of massive amounts of catecholamine into the blood stream can occur, a reaction known from other situations of stress.

This results in a hypertensive crisis. A critical drop in blood pressure is a much more unusual, but more serious incident. Angiographic procedures requiring selective CM administration should only be performed in pheochromocytoma patients after adequate treatment with alpha-adrenergic receptor blockers for a sufficient length of time (10-14 days).

## Sickle-cell anemia

In sickle-cell anemia patients, some erythrocytes contain the abnormal hemoglobin S. If $O_2$ pressure is lowered or blood osmolality is raised, HbS-containing blood corpuscles become inelastic and stretched. These erythrocytes can no longer pass through capillaries as easily, which can lead to stasis and to different forms of organ damage.

Administering high-osmolar CM to such patients is not without problems. The risk is highest for intra-arterial CM injection, especially in high doses, as is the case in cerebral and cardiac arteriography. In vitro studies comparing the effect of ionic and nonionic CM in terms of sickle-shaped changes of erythrocytes reveal that these changes are significantly less pronounced when nonionic CM is used [105].

# DRUGS AND MEASURES FOR THE TREATMENT OF A CONTRAST MEDIUM REACTION

A major prerequisite for using CM is a constant pre-paredness for the treatment of CM reactions. This includes the availability of trained medical personnel, the necessary equipment and appropriate drugs. Current recommendations for treating CM reactions are compiled in table 19.

A similar compilation was published by Bush and Swanson [106]. CM reactions have become very rare with the new, nonionic preparations; however, the need to be prepared for their treatment should never be neglected. One easily overlooked aspect is the expiry date on the preparations to be used for the treatment of such reactions.


U. Speck, *X-Ray Contrast Media*, https://doi.org/10.1007/978-3-662-56465-3_11

# Notes on the prophylaxis and therapy of X-ray contrast medium adverse effects

**Compiled by:**
Prof. Dr. Henrik S. Thomsen
Department of Diagnostic Radiology, Copenhagen
University Hospital at Herlev
Herlev Ringvej 75, DK-2730 Herlev, Denmark

**Updated by**
Prof. Dr. Martin Möckel
Department of Cardiology
Division of Emergency Medicine
Charité – Universitätsmedizin Berlin
Charitéplatz 1, 10711 Berlin, Germany
2016

**Precautions for a contrast medium injection are:**

- Explain to the patient about the examination and risk

- Create an anxiety-free examination atmosphere

- Ensure that first-line drugs and instruments are available

- Make sure that the patient is well hydrated

- Determine whether the patient is at risk of any contrast medium reaction

- Patients at risk should be carefully monitored during the examination

- When absorption or leakage into the circulation is possible (for example after intracavitar use), take the same precautions as for intravascular administration

| Adverse reaction | Risk factors / Conditions |
|---|---|
| **Previous generalised contrast medium reaction** | • Previous adverse reaction, either moderate (e.g. urticaria, bronchospasm, moderate hypotension) or severe (e.g. convulsions, severe bronchospam, pulmonary oedema, cardiovascular collapse) – anaphylactoid reactions<br>• Asthma<br>• Allergy requiring medical treatment |
| **Contrast medium induced nephrotoxicity** | • Raised s-creatinine levels, particularly secondary to diabetic nephropathy<br>• Dehydration<br>• Congestive heart failure<br>• Concurrent administration of nephrotoxic drugs, e.g. non-steroid<br>• anti-inflammatory drugs<br>• Age over 70 years old |
| **Lactic acidosis** | Patients treated with biguanide-type antidiabetics |
| **Anxiety** | Nervousness, sweating etc. |
| **Iodine induced hyperthyroidism** | • Patients with Graves' disease<br>• Multinodular goiter with thyroid autonomy, especially elderly patients and patients living in areas of iodine deficiency |
| **Extravasation** | • Power injector with insufficient fixation of needle placement<br>• Fragile or damaged veins<br>• Malposition of sheath or catheter |
| **Risk for late reaction (1 hour to 7 days)** | • Previous contrast medium reaction<br>• Interleukin-2 treatment |
| **Hypotension** | Dehydration |

* For complete information about possible risk factors, please refer to package-inserts, textbooks on contrast media or ESC / ESUR-guidelines for instance.

**Table. 19.** Recommendations for treating contrast media reactions

- Nonionic, low osmolal contrast media should be standard and the only one given under these circumstances
- Corticosteriods may be given:
  Prednisolone 30 mg orally 2 hours or Methylprednisolone 32 mg orally 12 and 2 hours before contrast medium; in case of urgency up to 250 mg Methylprednisolone may be given i.v.; solid data are lacking, therefore individual considerations need to be taken into account (e.g. severity of previous reactions)
- Effects of antihistamines [H1 and H2] are not definitely proven, but mostly used in clinical practise

- Make sure that the patients is well hydrated [give at least 100 mL (oral, e.g. soft drinks) or intravenous (normal saline) depending on the clinical situation) per hour starting 12 (at least 4 hours) before to 12 hours after contrast administration – in warm areas increase the fluid volume]
- Use nonionic, low osmolal contrast media
- Stop administration of nephrotoxic drugs for at least 24 hours
- Consider alternative imaging techniques, which do not require the administration of iodinated contrast media

- S-creatinine level measurement < 1 week
- S-creatinine normal
  - Stop biguanide intake, give contrast medium
- S-creatinine abnormal
  - Consider alternative imaging techniques, which do not require the administration of iodinated contrast media
  - Stop biguanide intake, postpone contrast medium examination 48 hours

- Talk to the patient, try to generate a positive, low-stress atmosphere;
- Consider benzodiazepines only if non-pharmacolic measures do not work

- Contrast media exposure should be limited to emergency procedures;
  - in these cases thyreostatic therapy needs to be initiated before contrast media (CM) exposure and iodine uptake needs to be blocked by Natriumperchlorat;
  - in all other cases diagnostics and treatment of hyperthyreoidism needs to come first and the examination using contrast media has to be delayed until thyroid hormones returned to normal

- Appropriate injection site, careful injection with use of appropriate sized cannula
- Prefer nonionic contrast medium in combination with power injector

Patient should be informed and observed

Hydrate adequately

The table only lists measures to be taken by attending physicians; if needed, additional treatment should be  left to a resuscitation team.

General: All patients in whom intravascular iodinated contrast medium administration is planned should have a tested venous line prior to the start of the examination.

| Acute adverse reactions (<1 hour) | |
| --- | --- |
| **Nausea/Vomiting** | **Moderate, transient:** Supportive treatment<br>**Severe, protracted:** Appropriate antiemetic drugs (e.g. odansetron, dimenhydrinat*) should be considered |
| **Urticaria** | **Scattered, transient:** Supportive treatment including observation<br>**Scattered, protracted:** Appropriate H1-antihistamine (e.g. clemastine*) preferably intravenously (intramusculary if no other option and timely treatment needed) should be considered. Drowsiness and/or hypotension may occur.<br>**Profound:** Consider Adrenaline 1:1000, 0.1–0.3 mL (0.1–0.3 mg) intravenously in adults, 0.01 mg/kg intravenously up to 0.3 max. in children. Repeat as needed. Alternative routes are intramuscular or intraossery, if no intravenous line is in function. |
| **Bronchospasm** | 1. Oxygen by mask (6–10 l/min)<br>2. ß-2-agonist metered dose inhaler, 2–3 deep inhalations (e.g. salbutamol*)<br>3. Adrenaline intravenously dependent on blood pressure and severity<br>    **Normal blood pressure**<br>        1:1000, 0.1–0.3 mL (0.1–0.3 mg) [use smaller dose in a patient with coronary artery disease or elderly patient],<br>        in children: 0.01 mg/kg; max dosage: 0.3 mg<br>    **Decreased blood pressure** (< 90 mmHg systolic)<br>        1:1000, 0.5 mL (0.5 mg), in children: 0.01 mg/kg, max. dosage: 0.3 mg<br>4. Intravenous bolus of corticosteroid, e.g. Prednisolon, 250 mg<br>5. For further treatment: resuscitation team |
| **Laryngeal edema** | 1. Oxygen by mask (6–10 l/min)<br>2. Intravenous adrenaline (1:1000), 0.1–0.3 mL (0.1–0.3 mg) for adults, repeat as needed<br>3. Intubation via resuscitation team<br>4. Intravenous bolus of corticosteroid, e.g. Prednisolon, 250 mg |
| **Hypotension** | **Isolated hypotension**<br>1. Elevate patient's legs<br>2. Oxygen by mask (6–10 l/min)<br>3. Intravenous fluid: rapidly, normal saline or lactated Ringer's solution<br>4. If unresponsive: adrenaline: 1:1000 , 0.1–0.3 mL (0.1–0.3 mg) intravenously, repeat as needed<br>**Vagal reaction (hypotension and bradycardia)**<br>1. Elevate patient's legs<br>2. Oxygen by mask (6–10 l/min)<br>3. Atropine 0.5–1.0 mg intravenously, repeat if necessary after 3–5 min, to 3 mg total (0.04 mg/kg) in adults, in pediatric patients give 0.02 mg/kg intravenously (max. 0.6 mg per dose) repeat if necessary to 2 mg total<br>4. Intravenous fluids: rapidly, normal saline or lactated Ringer's solution<br>**Hypotension and tachycardia**<br>1. Elevate patient's legs<br>2. Intravenous fluids: rapidly, normal saline or lactated Ringer's solution<br>3. Oxygen by mask (6–10 L/min) |
| **Anaphylactoid generalized reaction** | 1. Call for resuscitation team<br>2. Suction of airways as needed<br>3. Elevate patient's legs if hypotensive<br>4. Oxygen by mask (6–10 l/min)<br>5. Intravenous adrenaline (1:1000), 0.1–0.3 mL (0.1–0.3 mg) in adults. Repeat as needed. In pediatric patients 0.01 mg/kg to 0.3 mg max. dose<br>6. Intravenous fluids rapidly (e.g. normal saline, lactated Ringer's)<br>7. Intravenous bolus of corticosteroid, e.g. Prednisolon, 250 mg<br>8. H1-blocker e.g. diphenhydramine* 25–50 mg intravenously |
| **Seizures, Convulsions** | Diazepam* 5–10 mg rectally (or intravenously); or alternative (if available): Lorazepam, 2 mg |

**Table. 19.** Continuation

<table>
<tr><td colspan="2">Late adverse reactions (1 hour to 7 days)</td></tr>
<tr><td colspan="2">Symptomatic and similar to the management of other drug-induced skin reactions</td></tr>
<tr><td>Extravasation</td><td>• Conservative management is adequate in most cases<br>  – limb elevation<br>  – apply ice packs<br>  – careful monitoring<br>• If a serious injury is suspected, seek the advice of a surgeon</td></tr>
<tr><td>Iodine induced hyperthyroidism</td><td>• Very late reaction (several days/weeks)<br>• Seek the advice of an endocrinologist</td></tr>
<tr><td>Contrast medium induced nephrotoxicity</td><td>• Symptomatic<br>• Close monitoring as in any other patient with reduced renal function (due to other causes) – Consult a nephrologist<br>• Dialysis seems to have no effect on the incidence on contrast media induced nephropathy</td></tr>
<tr><td>Lactic acidosis</td><td>• Monitor renal function (serum creatinine), serum lactic acid and pH of blood<br>• Look for symptoms of lactic acidosis (vomiting, somnolence, nausea, epigastric pain, anorexia, hyperpnea, lethargy, diarrhea and thirst). Blood test results indicative of lactic acidosis: pH $< 7.25$ and lactic acid $> 5$ mmol</td></tr>
</table>

* The drugs available may vary from country to country.

**Table. 19.** Continuation

Keep in mind that even a "harmless" reaction e.g. nausea may result in an anaphylactoid generalized reaction. Every patient should always be kept under supervision during and right after contrast medium injection. High-risk patients should be monitored longer than low-risk patients.

# FURTHER DEVELOPMENT OF CONTRAST MEDIA

The development of CM aims at further improvement of tolerance and identification of new diagnostic options by altering pharmacokinetic properties. New technical developments of imaging modalities also influence the use of and need for CM with special properties.

It is expected that established state-of-the-art radiological techniques will be developed further, expanding current uses towards the examination of larger volumes, more rapid sequences, and lower radiation exposure. The standard radiological methods will retain their current role.

It will be hard to surpass the level of efficacy, tolerance and safety of current contrast media while simultaneously keeping the cost of products at an acceptable level.

© The Author(s) 2018

U. Speck, *X-Ray Contrast Media*, https://doi.org/10.1007/978-3-662-56465-3_12

New approaches in X-ray contrast medium research have evolved from studies with metal ion chelates for magnetic resonance imaging [107]. Heavy elements absorb X-rays more effectively than iodine but are much more difficult to bind to organic, well-tolerated and excretable substances in a suitable form. Initial clinical applications suggest the suitability of chelates for X-ray techniques but safety issues remain to be solved [108, 109].

New technical developments will further expand and modify the diagnostic possibilities in the years to come. Dynamic, physiologically controlled and high-resolution scanners improve detail resolution in CT, and very fast scanners allowing coverage of very large volumes with very short scan times are currently being introduced into clinical practice.

With the rapid infusion of well-tolerated CM, even better information on tissue perfusion, capillary permeability and the extracellular space of tissues can be obtained.

# REFERENCES


1. Gelfand DW. High-density low viscosity barium for fine mucosal detail on double-contrast upper gastrointestinal examinations. AJR 130(1978):831–833

2. Choi BI, Park JH, Kim BH, Kim SH, Han MC, Kim C-W. Small hepatocellular carcinoma: detection with sonography, computed tomography (CT), angiography and Lipiodol-CT. The British Journal of Radiology 62(1989):897–903

3. Almén T. Contrast agent design. Some aspects on the synthesis of water- soluble contrast agents of low osmolality. J Theor Biol 24(1969):216–226

4. Eichmann P. Der Vorteil der Amipaque - Urographie bei Risikopatienten. Urologe (B)22(1982):21–24

5. Rapoport S, Bookstein JJ, Higgins ChB, Carey PH, Sovak M, Lasser EC. Experience with metrizamide in patients with previous severe anaphylactoid reactions to ionic contrast agents. Radiology 143(1982):321–325

6. Katayama H, Yamaguchi K, Kozuka T, Takashima T, Seez P, Matsuura K. Adverse reactions to ionic and non-ionic contrast media. Radiology 175(1990):621–628

7. Wolf G, Arenson R, Cross A. A prospective trial of ionic versus nonionic contrast agents in routine clinical practice: Comparison of adverse effects. AJR 15 2,5(1989):939–944

8. Morcos SK, Thomsen HS. Adverse reactions to iodinated contrast media. Eur Radiol 11(2001):1267–1275

9. Palkowitsch PK, Bostelmann S, Lengsfeld P. Safety and tolerability of iopromide intravascular use;a pooled analysis of three non-interventional studies in 132,012 patients. Acta Radiol 55(2014):707–714

10. Krause W, Miklautz H, Kollenkirchen U, Heimann G. Physicochemical parameters of x-ray contrast media. Invest Radiol 29(1994):72–80

11. Speck U, Mützel W, Weinmann H-J. Chemistry, physiochemistry, and pharmacology of known and new contrast media for angiography, urography and CT enhancement; in Taenzer V, Zeitler E (eds), Contrast media in urography, angiography, and computerized tomography, pp 2–10 (Thieme, Stuttgart 1983)



© The Author(s) 2018

U. Speck, *X-Ray Contrast Media*, https://doi.org/10.1007/978-3-662-56465-3

12. Wolf K-J, Steidle B, Banzer D, Seyferth W, Keysser R. Comparative evaluation of low osmolar contrast media in (femoral) arteriography; in Taenzer V, Zeitler E (eds), Contrast media in urography, angiography and computerized tomography, pp 102–106 (Thieme, Stuttgart 1983)

13. Thron A, Ratzka M, Voigt K, Nadjmi M. Iohexol and ioxaglate in cerebral angiography; in Taenzer V, Zeitler E (eds), Contrast media in urography, angiography, and computerized tomography, pp 115–119 (Thieme, Stuttgart 1983)

14. Knoefel PK, Kraft RP, Knight RD, Moore SK. Sodium versus meglumine diatrizoate in excretory urography. Invest Radiol 9(1974):117–12

15. Taenzer V, Koeppe R, Samwer KF, Kolb GH. Comparative pharmacokinetics of sodium- and methylgluycamine-diatrizote in urography. Europ J clin Pharmacol 6 (1973):137–140

16. Steger-Hartmann T, Länge R, Schweinfurth H. Environmental risk assessment for the widely used iodinated x-ray contrast agent iopromide (Ultravist). Ecotoxicology and Environmental Safety 42(1999):274–281

17. Hughes PM, Bisset R. Nonionic contrast media: a comparison of iodine delivery rates during manual injection angiography. Brit J Radiol 64(1991):417–419

18. Felder E, Zingales MF, Tiepolo U. Radiopaque contrast media. XLVII-Iopamidol: Proposed analytical monograph. Boll Chim Farm 120(1981):639–648

19. Felder E. Pharmaceutical-chemical considerations related to the safety of nonionic X-ray contrast agents. Invest Radiol 19 Suppl 4(1984):145

20. Wang Y-CJ. Deiodination kinetics of water-soluble radiopaques. J Pharm Sci 69(1980):671–675

21. Morris TW, Sahler LG, Fischer HW. Calcium binding by radiopaque media. Invest Radiol 17(1982):501–505

22. Winding O. Intrinsic particles in angiographic contrast media. Radiology 134(1980):317–320

23. Fischer HW. Contamination of contrast agents by rubber components of 50 ml disposable syringes. Radiology 152(1984):540 (Commentary)

24. Dawson P, Becker A, Holton JM. The effect of contrast media on the growth of bacteria. Brit J Radiol 56(1983):809–815

25. Hamilton G. Contamination of contrast agents by rubber components of 50 ml disposable syringes. Radiology 152(1984):539–540

26. Blake MP, Halasz SJ. The effects of x-ray contrast media on bacterial growth. Australasian Radiology 39(1995):10–13

27. Tress BM, Hellyar AG, Pennington J, Thomson KR, Martinkus J, Lavan JJ. Bacteriological studies of open versus closed contrast medium delivery systems in angiography. Australasian Radiology 38(1994):112–114

28. Taenzer V, Speck U, Wolf R. Pharmakokinetik und Plasmaeiweißbindung von Iotroxinsäure (Biliscopin), Iodoxaminsäure (Endomirabil) und Ioglycaminsäure (Biligram). Röfo 126(1977):262–267

29. Krause W, Niehues D. Biochemical characterization of x-ray contrast media. Invest Radiol 31(1996):30–42

30. Dawson P, Turner MW, Bradshaw A, Westaby S. Complement activation and generation of C3a anaphylatoxin by radiological contrast agents. Brit J Radiol 56(1983):447–448

31. Vieluf D, Ring J. Anaphylaktoide Reaktionen durch Röntgenkontrastmittel. In: Peters PE, Zeitler E (eds): Röntgenkontrastmittel, Nebenwirkungen, Prophylaxe, Therapie. Springer-Verlag, Berlin-Heidelberg-New York, (1991):83–95

32. Krause W. Preclinical characterization of iopromide. Invest Radiol 29(1994):21–32

33. Lasser EC, Lyon SG. Inhibition of angiotensin-converting enzyme by contrast media: in vitro findings. Invest Radiol 25(1990):698–702

34. Lasser EC. Metabolic basis of contrast material. Toxicity-status. AJR 113(1971):415–422

35. Kimball JP. Red blood cell aggregation versus blood clot formation in ionic and non-ionic contrast media. Invest Radiol 23(1988):334–339

36. Hoffmann JJML, Tielbeek AV, Krause W. Haemostatic effects of low osmolar non-ionic and ionic contrast media: a double-blind comparative study. The British Institute of Radiology 73(2000):248–255

37. Chonos NAF, Goodall AH, Wilson DJ, Sigwart U, Buller NP. Profound platelet degranulation is an important side effect of some types of contrast media used in interventional cardiology. Circulation 88(1993):2035–2044

38. Jung F, Spitzer SG, Pindur G. Effect of an ionic compared to a non-ionic x-ray contrast agent on platelets and coagulation during diagnostic cardiac catheterization Pathopysiol Haemost Thromb 32(2002):121–126

39. Krause W, Press WR. Influence of contrast media on blood coagulation. Invest Radiol 32(1997):249–259

40. Jones CI, Goodall AH. Differential effects of the iodinated contrast agents ioxaglate, iohexol and iodixanol on thrombus formation and fibrinolysis. Thrombosis Research 112(2003):65–71

41. Rasuli P, McLeish WA, Hammond DI. Anticoagulant effects of contrast materials: in vitro study of iohexol, ioxaglate, and diatrizoate. AJR 152(1989):309–311

42. Saito M, Itoth Y, Yano T, Sendo T, Goromaru T, Sakai N, Oishi R. Roles of intracellular Ca(2+) and cyclic AMP in mast cell histamine release induced by radiographic contrast media. Naunyn -Schmiedebergs Archives of Pharmacology 367(2003):364–371

43. Battenfeld R, Rahman Khater AE, Drommer W, Guenzel P, Kaup FJ. Ioxaglate-induced light and electron microscopic alterations in the renal proximal tubular epithelium of rats. Invest Radiol 26(1991):35–39

44. Dawson P. Cardiovascular effects of contrast agents. Am J Cardiol 64(1989):2E–9E

45. Nyman U, Almen T, Landtman M. Effect of pH, buffer and osmolality of different contrast media on aortic blood pressure in the rabbit. Acta Radiol Diagnosis 21(1980):Fasc 5

46. Donadio C, Tramonti G, Lucchesi A, Giordani R, Lucchetti A, Bianchi C. Tubular toxicity is the main renal effect of contrast media. Renal Failure 18(1996):647–656

47. Liss P. Effect of contrast media on renal microcirculation and oxygen tension. An experimental study in the rat. Acta Radiologica 409(1997):7–29

48. Barrett BJ, Carlisle EJ. Metaanalysis of the relative nephrotoxicity of high and low osmolality iodinated contrast media. Radiology 188(1993):171–178

49. Marenzi G, Lauri G, Assanelli E. Contrast-induced nephropathy in patients undergoing primary angioplasty for acute myocardial infarction. J Am Coll Cardiol 44(2004):1780–1785

50. Morcos SK, Thomson HS, Webb JW. Contrast media induced nephrotoxicity; a consensus report. Eur Radiol 9(1999):1602–1613

51. Thomsen HS, Morcos SK. Contrast media Safety Committee of European Society of Urogenital Radiology. Management of acute adverse reactions to contrast media. Eur Radiol 14(2004):476–448

52. Laroche D, Aimone-Gastin I, Dubois F. Mechanism of severe, immediate reactions to iodinated contrast material. Radiology 209(1989):183–190

53. Dewachter P, Laroche D, Mouton-Faivre C, Clemont O. Immediate and late adverse reactions to iodinated contrast media: a pharmacological point of view. Anti-inflammatory antiallergy agents. Med Chem 5(2006):105–117

54. Christiansen C. Late-onset allergy-like reactions to x-ray contrast media. Curr Opin Allergy Clin Immunol 2(2002):533–539

55. Schild HH, Kuhl CK, Hübner-Steiner U, Böhm I, Speck U. Adverse events after unenhanced and monomeric and dimeric contrast-enhanced CT: a prospective randomized controlled trial. Radiology 240 (2006):56–64

56. Webb JAW, Stacul E, Thomsen HS, Morcos DK. Late adverse reactions to intravascular iodinated contrast media. Eur Radiol 13(2003):181–184

57. Brockow K, Christiansen C, Kanny G et al. Management of hypersensitivity reactions to iodinated contrast media. Allergy 60(2005):150–158

58. Zhang H, Holt CM, Malik N. Effects of radiographic contrast media on proliferation and apoptosis of human vascular endothelial cells. Br J Radiol 73(2000):1034–1041

59. Bach R, Jung F, Scheller B, Hummel B, Özbek C, Spitzer S, Schieffer Influence of a non-ionic radiography contrast medium on the microcirculation. Acta Radiol 37(1996):214–217

60. McIvor, Steiner TJ, Perkin GD, Greenhalgh RM, Rose FC. Neurological morbidity of arch and carotid arteriography in cerebrovascular disease. The influence of contrast medium and radiologist. Br J Radiol 60(1987):117–122

61. Skalpe IO, Nakstad P. Myelography with iohexol (Omnipaque); a clinical report with special reference to the adverse effects. Neuroradiology 30(1988):169–174

62. Wilson AJ, Evill CA, Sage MR. Effects of nonionic contrast media on the blood-brain barrier: osmolality versus chemotoxicity. Invest Radiol 26(1991):1091–1094

63. Whisson CC, Evill CA, Sage MR, Wilson AJ. Effect of additional cations on the twitching reaction to intracarotid, nonionic contrast media in rabbits. Invest Radiol 25(1990):1004–1009

64. Clauss W, Speck U. Pharmakologische Eigenschaften jodierter Röntgenkontrastmittel. In: Peters PE, Zeitler E (eds): Röntgenkontrastmittel. Nebenwirkungen, Prophylaxe, Therapie. Springer-Verlag. Berlin-Heidelberg-New-York (1991):18–29

65. Conradi A, Menta R, Cambi V. Pharmacokinetics of iopamidol in adults with renal failure. Arzneimittelforschung/Drug Res 40II(1990):830–832

66. Morcos SK, Thomsen HS, Webb JW. Prevention of generalized reactions to contrast media: a consensus report and guidelines. Eur Radiol 11(2001):1720–1728

67. Sharma S, Rajani M, Khosla A, Misra N, Goulatia RK. The influence of Buscopan on adverse reactions to intravascular contrast media. Br J Radiol 62(1989):1056–1058

68. Gupta R. Use of intravenous contrast agents in patients receiving metformin. Radiology 225,1(2002):311–312

69. Thomsen HS, Morcos SK. In which patients should serum creatinine be measured before iodinated contrast medium administration? Eur Radiol 15(2005):749–754

70. Harnish PP, Morris TW, Fischer HW, King AN. Drugs providing protection from severe contrast media reactions. Invest Radiol 15(1980):248–259

71. Virkkunen P, Luostarinen M, Johansson G. Diazepam, alpha and beta neurotransmission modifying drugs and contrast media mortality in mice. Acta Radiol (Diag) 25(1984):249–251

72. Peck WW, Slutsky RA, Mancini GBJ, Higgins ChB. Combined actions of verapamil and contrast media on artrioventricular conduction. Invest Radiol 19(1984):202–207

73. Pallan TM, Wulkan IA, Abadir AR, Flores L, Chaudhry MR, Gintautas J. Incompatibility of Isovue 370 and papaverine in peripheral arteriography. Radiology 187(1993):257–259

74. Weinstein JM, Heymann S, Brezis M. Potential deleterious effect of furosemide in radiocontrast nephropathy. Nephron 62(1992):413–415

75. Maly P, Olivecrona H, Almén T, Golman K. Interaction between chlorpromazine and intrathecally injected non-ionic contrast media in non-anaesthetized rabbits. Neuroradiology 26(1984):235–240

76. Kim SH, Lee HK, Han MC. Incompatibility of water-soluble contrast media and intravascular pharmacologic agents. An in vitro study. Invest Radiol 27(1992):45–49

77. Irvin HD, Burbridge BE. Incompatibility of contrast agents with intravascular medications. Radiology 173(1989):91

78. Husted SE, Kanstrup H. Thrombotic complications in coronary angioplasty-ionic versus non-ionic low osmolar contrast media. Acta Radiologica 39(1998):340–343

79. Smith HJ, Jones K, Hunter TB. What happens to patients after upper and lower gastrointestinal tract barium studies? Invest Radiol 23(1988):822–826

80. Freczko PJ, Simms SM, Bakirci N. Fatal hypersensitivity reaction during a barium enema. AJR 153(1989):275–276

81. Shehadi WH, Toniolo G. Adverse reaction to contrast media. Radiology 137(1980):299–302

82. Schott KM, Behrends B, Clauß W, Kaufmann J, Lehnert J. Iohexol in der Ausscheidungsurographie. Fortschr Med 104(1986):153–156

83. Palmer FJ. The RACR survey of intravenous contrast media reactions final report. Australas Radiol 32(1989):426–428

84. Cochran ST, Bomyea K, Sayre JW. Trends in adverse events after IV administration of contrast media. AJR 176(2001):1385–1388

85. Delayed allergy-like reactions to x-ray contrast media. Insert in European Radiology 6(5)(1996):1–24

86. Sutton AGC, Finn P, Campbell PG, Price DJA, Hall JA, Stewart MJ, Davies A, Linker NJ, Harcombe AA, de Belder MA. Early and late reactions following the use of iopamidol 340, iomeprol 350 and iodixanol 320 in cardiac catheterization. J Invas Cardiol 15(2003):133–138

87. Ring J, Rothenberger K-H. Anaphylaktoide Reaktionen nach Infusion von Röntgenkontrastmitteln. Münch Med Wschr 126(1984):657–661

88. Wolf G, Arenson R, Cross A. A prospective trial of ionic versus non-ionic contrast agents in routine clinical practice: comparison of adverse effects. AJR 152(1989):939–944

89. Brismar J, Jacobsson BF, Jorulf H. Miscellaneous adverse effects of low-versus high-osmolality contrast media: A study revised. Radiology 179(1991):19–23

90. Holtås S. Iohexol in patients with previous adverse reactions to contrast media. Invest Radiol 19(1984):563–565

91. Lasser EC, Berry C, Talner L, Santini L, Lang E. (NSC-MR) – Preliminary communication Association of University Radiologists. 32nd Annual Meeting, Newport Beach, California, (1984)

92. Reimann H-J, Tauber R, Kramann B, Gmeinwieser J, Schmidt U, Reiser M. Prämedikation mit H1- und H2-Rezeptorantagonisten vor intravenöser Kontrastmitteldarstellung der ableitenden Harnwege. Fortschr Röntgenstr 144(1986):169–173

93. Lasser EC, Berry CC, Mishkin MM, Williamson B, Zheutlin N, Silverman JM. Pretreatment with corticosteroids to prevent adverse reactions to nonionic contrast media. AJR 162(1994):523–526

94. Fink U, Jung D, Fink BK. Prämedikation bei Risikopatienten – Ergebnisse einer prospektiven Studie mit nichtionischen Kontrastmitteln; in Peters PE, Zeitler E (Hrsg) Röntgenkontrastmittel-Nebenwirkungen. Prophylaxe. Therapie, pp 205–209 (Springer, Berlin 1991)

95. Rendl J, Saller B. Schilddrüse und Röntgenkontrastmittel: Pathophysiologie, Häufigkeit und Prophylaxe der jodinduzierten Hyperthyreose. Dtsch Ärztebl 98(2001):316–320

96. Cramer BC, Parfrey PS, Hutchinson AT, Baran D, Melanson DM, Ethier RE, Seely IF. Renal function following infusion of radiologic contrast material. A prospective controlled study. Arch Intern Med 145(1985):87–89

97. Heller CA, Knapp J, Halliday J, O'Connell D, Heller RF. Failure to demonstrate contrast nephrotoxicity. Med J Aust 155(1991):329–332

98. Katzberg RW, Newhouse JH. Intravenous contrast medium-induced nephrotoxity: is the risk really as great as we have come to believe? Radiology 256(2010):21–28

99. Davenport MS, Khalatbari S, Cohan R, Dillman JR, Myles JD, Ellis JH. Contrast material-induced nephrotoxicity and intravenous low-osmolality iodinated contrast material: risk stratification by using estimated glomerular filtration rate. Radiology 268(2013):719–728

100. Solomon RJ, Natarajan MK, Doucet S, Sharma SK, Staniloae CS, Katholi E, Gelormini JL, Labinanz M, Moreyra AE. Cardiac angiography in renally impaired patients (care) study a randomized double-blind trial of contrast-induced nephropaphy in patients with chronic kidney disease. Circulation 115(2007):3189–3196

101. Katzberg RW, Barett BJ. Risk of iodinated contrast material induced nephropathy with intravenous administration. Radiology 243(2007):622–628

102. McCarthy CS, Becker JA. Multiple myeloma and contrast media. Radiology 183(1992):519–521

103. Friedrichsohn CB, Riegel W, Köhler H. Was ist gesichert in der Prävention der Kontrastmittelnephropathie? Med Klin 92(1997):329–334

104. Katholi RE, Taylor GJ, McCann WP, Woods WT Jr, Womack KA, McCoy CD, Katholi CR, Moses HW, Moses HW, Mishkel GJ, Lucore CL. Nephrotoxicity from contrast media: attentuation with theophylline. Radiology 195(1995):17–22

105. Rao VM, Rao Ak, Steiner RM, Burka ER, Grainger RG, Ballas SK. The effect of ionic and nonionic contrast media on sickling phenomenon. Radiology 144(1982):291–293

106. Bush H, Swanson DP. Acute reactions to intravascular contrast media: Types, risk factors, recognition, and specific treatment. AJR 157(1991):1153–1161

107. Zwicker C, Langer M, Urich V, Felix R. Kontrastgebung von Jod, Gadolinium und Ytterbium in der CT. Fortschr Röntgenstr 158(1993):255–259

108. Quinn AD, O'Hare NJ, Wallis FJ, Wilson GF. Gd-DTPA: An alternative contrast medium CT. J Comput Assist Tomogr 18(1994):634–636

109. Schild HH, Weber W, Boeck E, Mildenberger P, Strunk H, Düber C, Grebe P, Schadman-Fischer S, Thelen M. Gadolinium-DTPA (Magnevist) als Kontrastmittel für die arterielle DSA. Fortschr Röntgenstr 160(1994):218–221